Renal Glomerular Diseases

Renal Glomerular Diseases

Paul Sharpstone, FRCP

Consultant Physician,
Royal Sussex County Hospital, Brighton

and

J. A. P. Trafford, FRCP

Consultant Physician,
Royal Sussex County Hospital, Brighton

Published,
in association with
UPDATE PUBLICATIONS LTD., by

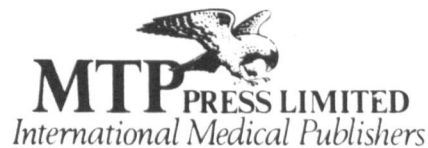

MTP PRESS LIMITED
International Medical Publishers

Published,
in association with
Update Publications Ltd., by

MTP Press Limited
Falcon House
Lancaster, England

Copyright © 1981 MTP Press Limited
Softcover reprint of the hardcover 1st edition 1981
First published 1981

ISBN-13: 978-94-009-8071-6   e-ISBN-13: 978-94-009-8069-3
DOI: 10.1007/978-94-009-8069-3

Contents

Note: Colour plates (1 to 22) can be found facing page 24

Preface

The cause of end-stage renal failure in one-third of patients treated by regular haemodialysis or kidney transplantation is some variety of glomerular disease. Less serious glomerular disorders are more common and often cause inappropriate consternation to the patients and, sometimes, to their doctors. Similar clinical features can be produced by pathological lesions ranging from the trivial to the life-threatening, and renal biopsy is often necessary to establish the diagnosis. However, its widespread use during the past 20 years has enabled clinicopathological correlations to be made and the natural history of many 'glomerulopathies' to be established, though large areas of uncertainty remain.

In contrast to symptomatic measures, such as the management of uraemia or the nephrotic syndrome, the use of treatment in arresting the progress of the glomerular lesion itself is controversial and is based on anecdotal evidence rather than controlled trials. Knowledge of the renal pathology will, at least, enable conditions in which immunosuppressive therapy is appropriate to be distinguished from those which are benign or self-limiting.

In this book symptomatic management of the clinical syndromes is detailed, but classification is firmly based on renal histological appearances. The relevance of immunofluorescent microscopy, ultrathin section examination and electron microscopy to our understanding of pathogenesis is described, as well as the uses of these techniques for morphological discrimination. Though we do not know the underlying cause of most varieties of glomerular disease, there is a wealth of information about the immunological pathogenesis of the lesions and the mediation of injury.

Renal Glomerular Diseases

A scheme for the investigation of patients with suspected glomerular disease, including measurement of renal function, is given. The technique of renal biopsy is described, and its indications, which are based on an appreciation of the possible pathological bases of the clinical syndrome with which the patient presents.

Paul Sharpstone
Royal Sussex
County Hospital, Brighton
January 1981

1. Introduction

There is glomerular damage in virtually every kidney disorder, but this monograph deals with those conditions characterized by primary involvement of the glomeruli. The term 'glomerulonephritis' is usually used, even though these disorders are not all inflammatory in nature. More accurate but less attractive alternatives such as 'primary glomerulopathy' do not seem to have been widely accepted.

The major problem is that of nomenclature. In other systems a single term, such as 'measles' or 'motor neurone disease', is often sufficient to define a disease even though its clinical features may be diverse or its aetiology unknown. Not so in nephrology, since, until recently, almost the only information available about renal histopathology was that obtained at autopsy, and the appearance of the end-stage kidney offered little clue to the pathology earlier in the course of the disease. The result was the construction of several eponymous classifications of nephritis, such as that of Ellis (1942), which were based on clinical rather than pathological features. These were invaluable in their time, but in the last 20 years the widespread use of kidney biopsy has revealed the diversity of renal glomerular pathology and made the older classifications less relevant. They will not be considered further here.

The correlation of clinical features with biopsy findings has elevated several renal glomerular disorders to the status of discrete 'diseases' with fairly well defined natural histories and pathological appearances. In some cases the clinical features are sufficiently characteristic to enable the pathology to be assumed without recourse to biopsy (for example acute post-streptococcal glomerulonephritis) but in many cases biopsy is necessary for a pathological diagnosis.

However, biopsy does not provide all the answers. Many renal histological appearances are non-specific in that they may be associated with a variety of clinical pictures. Conversely, most clinical syndromes may be due to a wide range of pathological lesions. For example, the pathologist examining a renal biopsy can never determine whether or not the patient has the nephrotic syndrome; and the histological appearance of the kidney of a patient with lupus nephritis cannot be predicted by the clinician. Further, the areas of our ignorance of aetiology are still wide, so that even when both the clinical features and renal pathology are known it may still be impossible to apply a single disease label to the patient's condition.

Nomenclature

Until our knowledge of nephrology improves, it is much more rational and helpful to avoid straight-jacket classifications, and to use a nomenclature which is purely descriptive. Unwarranted assumptions are avoided and nomenclature can be modified easily in the light of changing knowledge.

A complete diagnosis requires:

1. A description of the clinical features of the patient's disorder, i.e. the disturbance of function which brings him to medical attention.

2. The renal pathology, i.e. the disorder of structure which leads to the disordered function.

3. The aetiology, i.e. the cause of the structural disturbance.

This three-tier diagnosis will often have to be incomplete. The aetiology of most forms of glomerular disease is unknown, so the third tier will usually be omitted. If renal tissue has not been examined, or the pathology is assumed, the second tier cannot be completed.

It is important to be quite clear as to whether a term used refers to a pathological or a clinical feature. Much confusion has been caused in the past by the inappropriate use of terminology. For example, the term 'focal nephritis', which is a pathological description, has been applied to the clinical syndrome of recurrent haematuria; and 'sub-acute nephritis', a clinical syndrome, has been used to describe a particular histological appearance.

The three-tier diagnosis is widely used in fields of medicine other than nephrology. For example, in cardiology, a patient may have acute left ventricular failure (tier one) due to aortic incompetence (tier two) due to chronic rheumatic carditis (tier three). In liver medicine we have portosystemic encephalopathy due to hepatic cirrhosis due to alcoholism. Its use in nephrology, along with the acceptance that there is a lot left to learn, will make it much easier to make sense of nephritis.

2. Clinical Syndromes

Although the range of renal histopathology is enormous, the clinical expression of glomerular disease is limited. For example, uraemia caused by widespread obliteration of the glomeruli by amyloid is clinically and biochemically the same as that caused when a similar number of glomeruli are destroyed by membranous neuropathy. Thus there are relatively few clinical syndromes (Table 1) which may bring the patient with glomerular disease to medical attention. Most of them may be caused by a large number of pathological processes, and it is the latter which determine the prognosis.

The syndromes cannot be defined with precision, and a patient may present with features of more than one. Furthermore, different syndromes may occur in succession during the course of a single disease. Thus a patient may present with asymptomatic proteinuria, later become nephrotic, and ultimately die of chronic renal failure. Nevertheless, for a complete diagnosis it is necessary to specify the clinical features as well as the pathology, because it

Table 1. The clinical syndromes in renal glomerular disease.

Asymptomatic proteinuria
Recurrent isolated haematuria
Acute nephritic syndrome
Nephrotic syndrome
Acute renal failure
Chronic renal failure

is the functional disturbance which determines the patient's dis-
comfort. In addition, in the absence of effective treatment of the
renal lesion in the majority of cases, most therapeutic efforts are
directed towards the functional rather than the pathological disorder.

Asymptomatic Proteinuria

In asymptomatic proteinuria a patient with no symptoms refer-
able to the urinary tract is found to have protein in the urine at
routine examination (most commonly for life assurance, pre-
employment or military service). Subsequent investigation may
reveal other evidence of kidney disease, such as a raised blood
urea or red blood cells in the urine, but in many cases proteinuria
is the only manifestation.

An important variant is orthostatic proteinuria; this is the presence of protein in the urine after activity, but its absence after a
period of recumbency, such as before getting out of bed in the
morning.

Recurrent Isolated Haematuria

Recurrent isolated haematuria refers to macroscopic haematuria
in a patient who has no other clinical manifestation of renal
disease. Most of these patients are referred first to urological
surgeons, and with good reason, since often the cause will be
'surgical', e.g. a tumour of the bladder or kidney, or a urinary
calculus. Such conditions must always be excluded by pyelography
and cystoscopy before considering glomerular disease as the
cause. A distinction should be drawn between patients with
isolated haematuria and those with significant proteinuria as well.
The latter group generally have more serious underlying renal
lesions and a graver prognosis.

Isolated haematuria due to renal parenchymal disease is often
intermittent, and attacks may recur at intervals for many years.
They are often precipitated by upper respiratory tract infections
and may be confused with acute post-streptococcal nephritis.

However, the haematuria follows the infection immediately, not after an interval, and the infections are often viral rather than streptococcal. These infections are probably non-specific precipitating factors of the haematuria, and not the cause of the renal disease. The syndrome of recurrent isolated haematuria mostly affects children, but may occur at any age.

Acute Nephritic Syndrome

The clinical features of 'classical' acute nephritis are well known. The patient is most commonly a child of early school age, although the condition may occur at any age. The onset is acute with headache, malaise, anorexia, often pain in the back, and vomiting. Periorbital puffiness, swelling of the ankles, and dark or smoky urine are usual, and the patient or his parents may notice a reduction in urine volume.

A variety of glomerular diseases can present in this way, but post-streptococcal nephritis is the most common.

Post-streptococcal Nephritis

A streptococcal infection precedes the onset of the nephritis by one to three weeks. Usually this infection is tonsillitis or pharyngitis, but sometimes other sites, such as the middle ear or skin, may be involved. In contrast to rheumatic fever, only certain types, especially 12, 4, or 49 of the haemolytic Streptococcus group A, may be responsible. Between the infection and the renal disease there is usually a latent period, during which the patient feels quite well. When the disease is established, examination reveals periorbital and often generalized oedema, hypertension and the signs of circulatory overload with raised jugular venous pressure, a gallop rhythm and sometimes pulmonary crepitations.

Investigations show proteinuria, usually of moderate degree, haematuria, usually macroscopic, and many granular or red blood cell casts in the urine. The urine specific gravity is high and, in contrast to the oliguria of acute tubular necrosis, the urine sodium concentration is low (less than 40 mmol/l). The blood urea and creatinine may be raised but not usually by very much. Evidence of a recent streptococcal infection may be obtained by throat swab and by a raised ASO titre. However, the latter may be normal, particularly if the patient has been given antibiotics. The serum concentration of the third component of complement (C3) is usually reduced to below normal levels during the first few weeks of the illness. It must be emphasized that many patients do not show all of the classical features, and in some well-documented cases even proteinuria has been absent.

In most cases recovery is rapid. Oliguria persists for only a few days and, when diuresis occurs, hypertension, oedema and circulatory overload remit quickly. However, proteinuria and microscopic haematuria may persist for months or even years.

The complications of the disease are: heart failure, hypertensive encephalopathy with headache, drowsiness, vomiting, convulsions, sometimes focal neurological signs and ultimately coma, and persisting oliguria. Each of these may be fatal, but effective means of treatment are available for the first two, so that death is now rare from these causes. Oliguria persisting for more than a few days, however, usually signifies irreversible destruction of the glomeruli, so that recovery of useful renal function is unusual.

Outcome

Up-to-date figures are not available, but the mortality in the acute phase is very low and certainly much lower than one per cent.

Most patients recover rapidly from the acute attack, but a few develop a rapidly progressive form of the disease with increasing impairment of renal function, so that end stage renal failure develops within a few weeks or months. Persistent macroscopic haematuria and heavy proteinuria, as well as a rising blood urea and creatinine, characterize this variety of the disease, and many patients pass through a nephrotic phase. Older names for this condition are 'sub-acute nephritis' and nephritis with a 'stormy course'. Rapidly progressive glomerulonephritis, as it is usually called, is not rare and probably affects middle-aged and elderly patients more often than the young. In many instances good evidence of a streptococcal aetiology is lacking.

A more vexed question still is that of long-term prognosis in those patients who recover from the acute attack. It is often said that some 10 per cent of patients follow a slowly progressive course after acute nephritis. That is, they recover from the acute attack but enter a latent phase when proteinuria and perhaps microscopic haematuria persist. They remain clinically well for 10, 20 or more years, until features of renal failure and hypertension appear and lead ultimately to death. While some recent long-term follow-up studies of well documented post-streptococcal nephritis have demonstrated persistent disease, most have failed to demonstrate progression to renal failure, and it seems likely that few patients do follow a slowly progressive course. It is probable that many patients with progressive disease in the older series had a condition which would be diagnosed as something other than acute post-streptococcal nephritis by modern criteria. More long-term prospective studies are needed before the question is fully answered, but in the meantime it is important to give a good prognosis to patients who have recovered from typical acute post-streptococcal nephritis and whose renal function is normal. In the past too many patients have been rejected from certain occupations, or refused life insurance, or even made into chronic invalids without sufficient justification.

Nephrotic Syndrome

The nephrotic syndrome occurs when proteinuria is sufficiently heavy and prolonged to lead to hypoproteinaemia severe enough to cause oedema. The diagnosis is based on these features only and not on any arbitrary level of protein excretion or serum albumin. In practice the nephrotic syndrome rarely occurs unless the protein excretion is greater than 3 g/24 hr, and usually 5–10 g/24 hr or even higher protein excretion is needed to produce sufficient depletion of serum albumin (usually less than 30 g/l) to lead to oedema. Young patients, whose ability to synthesize albumin is greater than the elderly, may tolerate a protein loss of more than 10 g/24 hr for long periods without developing oedema.

Although there are many causes of proteinuria, the nephrotic syndrome is virtually always due to increased glomerular capillary permeability. Proteinuria from causes other than glomerular disease is rarely severe enough to cause the nephrotic syndrome.

The pathogenesis of the oedema (Figure 1) is not entirely clear. The initiating factor is the reduction in plasma colloid pressure, leading to increased transudation of intravascular fluid across the capillary wall into the interstitial fluid. The reduced intravascular volume activates the renin–angiotensin system to stimulate aldosterone secretion by the adrenal cortex. Aldosterone promotes sodium retention at the distal tubule and hence tends to correct the intravascular volume. Transudation continues across capillary walls and gradually there is sufficient interstitial fluid excess to produce clinically detectable oedema.

This is unlikely to be the whole story, however, and probably a reduction in glomerular filtration rate and other factors also operate to produce salt and water retention by the kidney. Nephrotic

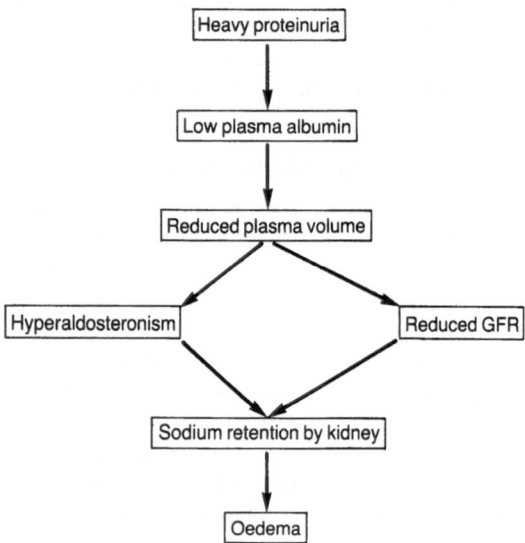

Figure 1. *Pathophysiology of the nephrotic syndrome.*

oedema tends to be less dependent in distribution than oedema of cardiac origin though this may be simply because nephrotic patients do not usually have pulmonary oedema and can lie flat in bed. The periorbital regions and hands are often affected, as well as the legs and sacrum. In extreme cases oedema may be generalized, and there may be ascites and pleural effusions as well.

Most nephrotic patients have an abnormality of plasma lipids, with hypercholesterolaemia and hypertriglyceridaemia. Its cause is unknown and its presence is by no means essential for the diagnosis of nephrotic syndrome.

Patients with the nephrotic syndrome may or may not have other manifestations of renal disease, such as uraemia, hypertension, haematuria or casts in the urine. These features depend entirely on the nature of the underlying renal lesion, as does the course and prognosis of the condition.

Complications peculiar to the nephrotic syndrome itself are seen less commonly now that powerful diuretics enable oedema to be controlled in most cases. Complications include cellulitis, pneumonia, peritonitis and other infections, muscle wasting, and venous thrombosis, including thrombosis of the renal vein. Serious complications may result from the depletion of intravascular volume. Although in many cases the measured plasma volume is within the normal range, nephrotic patients are most sensitive to depletion by, for example, diuretics, which may cause postural hypotension, sometimes hypovolaemic shock, and even tubular necrosis.

Acute Renal Failure

Acute renal failure is the abrupt cessation or severe impairment of renal function, usually but not invariably associated with oliguria (urine output less than 400 ml/24 hr in an adult). The clinical features are those of acute uraemia and of fluid and electrolyte overload. Acute renal failure is less often due to glomerular disease than to other conditions, especially acute tubular necrosis. This condition is described in another title in this series: *Acute and Chronic Renal Failure* (Boulton-Jones, 1980).

Chronic Renal Failure

Glomerular disease is one of the more important causes of chronic renal failure. It is the underlying disorder in at least one third of the patients who are treated with maintenance haemodialysis or transplantation. The clinical features of uraemia are the same whatever the underlying cause. Chronic renal failure is described in detail in another title in this series: *Acute and Chronic Renal Failure* (Boulton-Jones, 1980).

3. Pathology

Histological Methods

Most of our knowledge of renal histopathology comes from biopsy rather than autopsy material. As well as providing information about earlier stages of the disease, biopsy enables the techniques of electron microscopy and immunofluorescent microscopy to be applied. Even with light microscopy a much clearer picture is obtained with biopsy than with tissue obtained at autopsy. Details of the technique and indications for renal biopsy are given later.

Light Microscopy

Sections for light microscopy are cut to a thickness of $2-4 \mu m$. This is rather thinner than is usual in histology but it enables the capillary walls and basement membranes to be assessed more accurately. The three stains used routinely are haematoxylin and eosin (H and E), periodic-acid–Schiff (PAS) and silver methenamine. With silver methenamine the basement membranes are impregnated with silver and high power ($\times 1,000$) light microscopy under oil immersion enables the basement membrane detail to be seen. Many other stains are used for special purposes, for example to demonstrate amyloid and fibrin.

Electron Microscopy

Electron microscopy is a valuable tool in renal histological research but technical complexity confines its routine use to specialized centres. It is not often necessary for clinical purposes, but where practicable it is useful to mount some of the biopsy material so that it is suitable for retrospective electron microscopic examination, should this prove to be desirable. For this the material must be fixed in a different medium to that used for light microscopy, and it should be embedded in epoxy resin rather than in paraffin wax.

Ultrathin Sections

A recent development is the use of resin-embedded ultrathin sections for examination by light microscopy. These sections are cut to a thickness of $0.5-1$ μm, which is thicker than that necessary for electron microscopy, but it enables much finer structure to be resolved by the high power of the light microscope than is otherwise possible. This technique confers some of the advantages of electron microscopy, but is more widely applicable.

Immunofluorescent Microscopy

Immunofluorescent microscopy is a method of visualizing immunoglobulins and other immunologically reactive substances within the kidney. Sections of fresh biopsy material are treated with an antibody to the substance under investigation, the antibody having been previously conjugated with fluorescein dye. The antibody unites with its antigen in the kidney to form a complex which includes the fluorescein (Figure 2). After washing away unbound antibody the section is examined under ultraviolet light. The sites of the antigen are then visualized as areas of fluorescence. Immunofluorescent microscopy is applicable to many antigenic substances, including the various immunoglobulins, fractions of complement, and fibrinogen.

Microanatomy of Normal Kidney and Interpretation of Renal Histopathology

Glomerulus

A glomerulus is essentially a network of capillaries situated within the urinary space of Bowman's capsule (Plates 1 to 3). The capillary tuft is formed by branching of the afferent arteriole, and union of the capillaries forms the efferent arteriole. The proximal

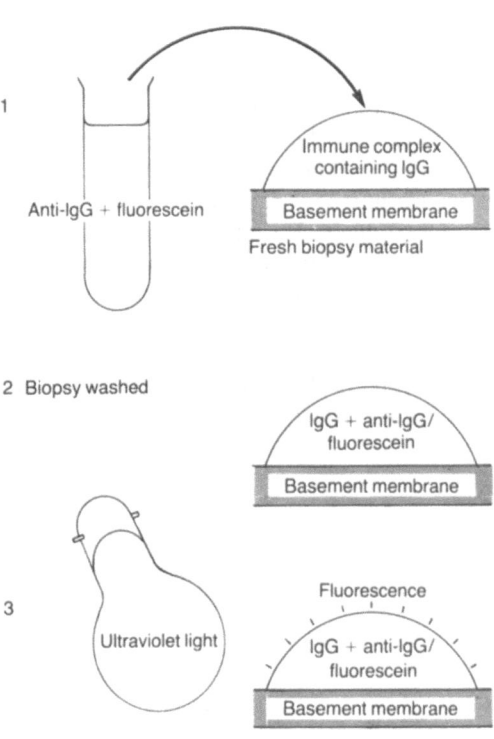

Figure 2. *Technique of immunofluorescent microscopy.*

convoluted tubule leads from Bowman's capsule so that the urinary space is continuous with the lumen of the tubule. Like capillaries elsewhere in the body the glomerular capillaries consist of basement membrane lined internally with endothelium and externally with epithelium. The capillary basement membrane is continuous at the hilum with that of Bowman's capsule and of the proximal tubule. Similarly, the capillary epithelium is continuous with the epithelium lining the inner surface of Bowman's capsule and the tubule. In the glomerular tuft the capillary loops are separated from each other by a small amount of ground substance, the mesangium, which contains the mesangial cells.

The finer structure of the capillary wall is discernible only with the electron microscope (Figure 3). The basement membrane is of fairly uniform thickness (about 12,000 nm), and has a central dense layer separating the inner and outer less dense layers. The endothelial cytoplasm is very thin, and like endothelium elsewhere has tiny fenestrations. The form of the epithelial cytoplasm, however, is unique to the glomerulus. It spreads from the nucleus, not as a continuous sheet, but as a number of radial processes known as foot processes, which themselves have multiple branches. Foot processes from adjacent cells interdigitate, so that in a transverse section of the capillary wall the epithelial cytoplasm has the form of a series of discrete masses separated by gaps

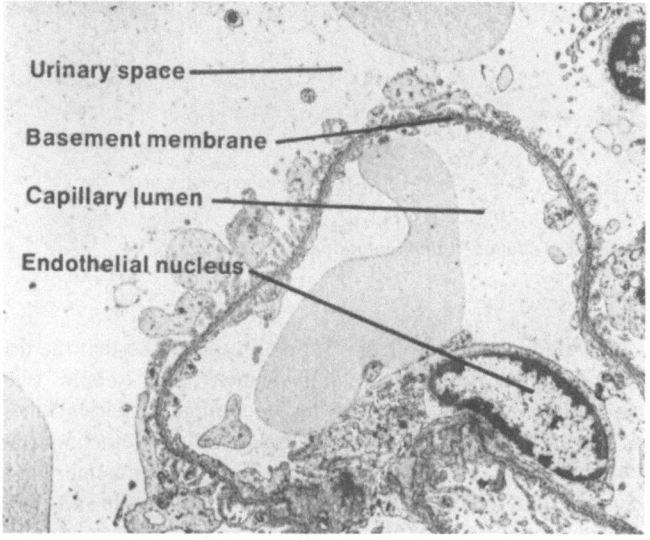

Figure 3. *Normal glomerulus, electron micrograph ×10,000.*

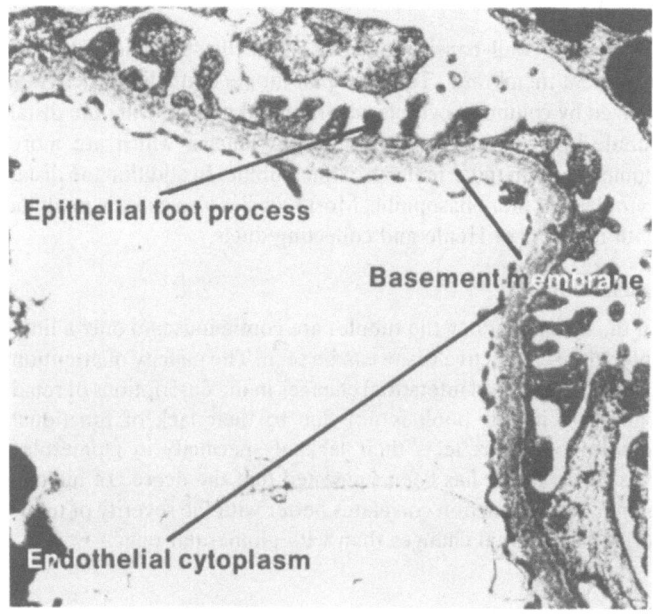

Figure 4. *Normal glomerulus, electron micrograph ×25,000.*

(Figure 4). The gaps between the foot processes are known as filtration slits, and are bridged over at the surface of the basement membrane by a thin membrane.

In the normal glomerulus stained with H and E and viewed with the light microscope (Plate 1) the capillaries can be seen as clear spaces containing red blood cells. The capillary wall, best seen at the periphery of the tuft, is thin, but details of its structure, such as the basement membrane, cannot be identified. A number of nuclei can be seen within the tuft but it is generally impossible to determine whether they are epithelial, endothelial or mesangial in nature. The mesangial cytoplasm, seen between the capillaries, is quite sparse.

Tubules

The tubule wall consists of epithelial cells surrounded by the basement membrane. The proximal tubule epithelium is characterized by columnar cytoplasm with basal nuclei, while the distal tubule has cuboidal cells with central nuclei, which are more numerous than those in the proximal tubule. In addition the distal cytoplasm is more basophilic. Most biopsies also contain medulla with its loops of Henle and collecting ducts.

Interstitium

In the normal kidney the tubules are contiguous and only a little interstitial connective tissue can be seen. The paucity of attention paid to tubular and interstitial changes in the descriptions of renal pathology in this book is not due to their lack of functional importance but reflects their lack of specificity in glomerular disease. In fact it has been suggested that the degree of impairment of renal function correlates better with the severity of tubular and interstitial changes than with glomerular ones.

Blood Vessels

Blood vessels ranging in size from capillary to interlobular can usually be found. Again the changes, though often functionally important, are rarely specific.

Assessment of Renal Histopathology

A systematic method of examining the renal biopsy should always be followed. After a general account of the adequacy of the specimen, especially the number of glomeruli, the above-mentioned structures should be looked at individually. Departures from the normal appearance in each case should be quantitated roughly, using such terms as 'mild', 'moderate' or 'severe'. Next, structures not present in the normal kidney, such as polymorphonuclear leucocytes in the glomerular tuft, amyloid deposits in the vessel walls, or chronic inflammatory cells in the interstitium, should be looked for. It is important to specify the distribution of glomerular lesions. If some of the glomeruli are affected by an abnormality and others are normal, the lesion is said to be focal. If only parts of glomeruli are involved, while the other areas of the same glomeruli are normal, it is said to be a segmental lesion.

Finally, it may be possible to summarize the histological findings with one of the diagnostic categories given in the next chapter. However, if doubt remains, it is much safer to detail the abnormalities found rather than to guess the diagnosis.

4. Pathological Appearances and Clinical Associations

Disorders in which the kidney is the only organ primarily involved by the disease process are considered separately from renal involvement in multisystem diseases. However, in many multisystem diseases the renal pathology may be indistinguishable from that in some of the primary conditions.

Primary Renal Disease

Five main varieties of primary renal disease (Table 2) are recognized on the basis of the histological appearances.

Proliferative Glomerulonephritis

Proliferative glomerulonephritis refers to a group of conditions with diverse histology, clinical features and aetiology, whose only common feature is an excess of cells (proliferation) in the glomeruli.

Table 2. Histological categories of primary glomerular disease.

Proliferative glomerulonephritis
   Diffuse proliferative exudative
   Mesangial proliferative
   Mesangiocapillary
   Focal proliferative
   Proliferative with extensive crescents

Membranous nephropathy

Minimal change disease

Focal hyalinosis

Unclassified glomerular lesions

Diffuse Proliferative Exudative Glomerulonephritis

Diffuse proliferative exudative glomerulonephritis is one of the specific pictures in renal histology (Plate 4). It is the hallmark of post-streptococcal acute glomerulonephritis. The glomeruli are swollen by proliferation of mesangial and endothelial cells and the capillary lumens are narrowed by this cellular excess, and by swelling of the endothelial cytoplasm. As a result there is a paucity of red blood cells in the capillary lumina. There is also an exudate of polymorphonuclear leucocytes in the capillaries and mesangial regions. In summary, there is an acute inflammation and ischaemia of the glomerulus. Immunofluorescent microscopy shows granular deposition of C3 and IgG along the capillary walls.

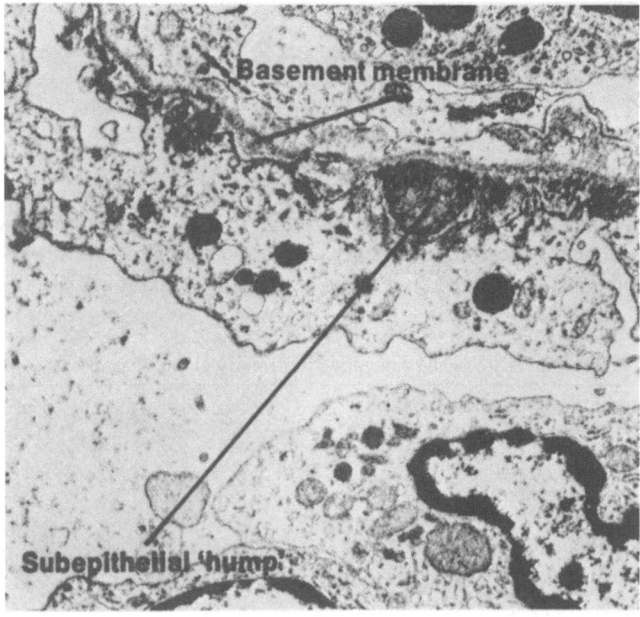

Figure 5. *Diffuse proliferative exudative glomerulonephritis, electron micrograph ×22,000.*

On electron microscopy a very characteristic feature is seen in the acute stage. This consists of nodules (often called 'humps') of electron-dense material on the outer surface of the basement membrane, separating it from the epithelial cytoplasm (Figure 5). The significance of these humps is considered in Chapter 5.

Despite the severity of the histological appearance the overall architecture of the glomerulus is not damaged, and complete or almost complete recovery takes place in the majority of cases within a few months. During the healing stage the most prominent residual feature is some hypercellularity in the mesangial areas of the lobules of the glomerular tufts. Minor changes, such as small areas of scarring and adhesions of the tuft to Bowman's capsule, may persist indefinitely, but are of little clinical significance.

Mesangial Proliferative Glomerulonephritis

In mesangial proliferative glomerulonephritis there is a hypercellularity in the central or axial regions of lobules due to proliferation of mesangial cells. There is also a variable increase of hyaline eosinophilic material in this region. When proliferation is inconspicuous the condition may be referred to as mesangial sclerosis.

These appearances are found in the healing phase of poststreptococcal glomerulonephritis as described above, but also in other clinical settings, such as the nephrotic syndrome, asymptomatic proteinuria or isolated haematuria. In these cases there is usually no evidence of a streptococcal aetiology. There is little or no impairment of renal function and the lesion does not appear to be a progressive one. Its natural history cannot be predicted with certainty in individual cases, but in general the prognosis is good. It is almost certainly of multifactorial aetiology.

Mesangiocapillary Glomerulonephritis

Mesangiocapillary glomerulonephritis is a term that has been introduced recently. It refers to a condition variously called in the older terminology 'chronic lobular', 'mixed membranous and proliferative', 'membranoproliferative', or 'persistent hypocomplementaemic nephritis'.

The salient histological feature is a combination of mesangial cell proliferation with thickening of the capillary wall (Plate 5). As well as hypercellularity in the lobular stalk region, there is an increase in the mesangial connective tissue, seen as a fibrillary appearance on PAS or silver stains. The lobular pattern of the glomerular tuft is often markedly accentuated.

Two types of capillary wall thickening are seen. In the majority of cases there is an invasion of endothelial cytoplasm by silver-staining fibrils similar to those in the mesangium. Condensation of these fibrils internal to the basement membrane leads to apparent reduplication of the membrane (Plate 6). Electron microscopy shows subendothelial deposits and immunofluorescence reveals granular deposition of Clq, C3 and IgG.

In the second and less common variety the capillary wall thickening is due to a 'ribbon-like', dense, linear deposit within the basement membrane itself (Plate 7). It is seen in the basement membranes of Bowman's capsule and tubules as well as the glomerular capillaries. The characteristic finding on immuno-fluorescent microscopy is the deposition of C3 but not of immunoglobulins.

When proliferation is inconspicuous the condition can be misdiagnosed as membranous nephropathy. However, the two conditions may be readily distinguished by examination of the morphology of the capillary wall in silver-stained preparations using the oil immersion objective, or by electron microscopy.

Mesangiocapillary glomerulonephritis mainly affects children of school age and young adults, and is slightly commoner in girls than boys. It may present as asymptomatic proteinuria, recurrent haematuria, the nephrotic syndrome, or as an acute nephritis-like illness. The last mode of presentation is very important, since the prognosis is far worse than that of post-streptococcal acute glomerulonephritis. It may be that the reported progressive course of a proportion of patients with post-streptococcal disease was due to the inclusion of cases of mesangiocapillary glomerulonephritis with an acute nephritic onset.

All patients have proteinuria, which may be heavy, and the majority have haematuria. About 50 per cent of the patients have

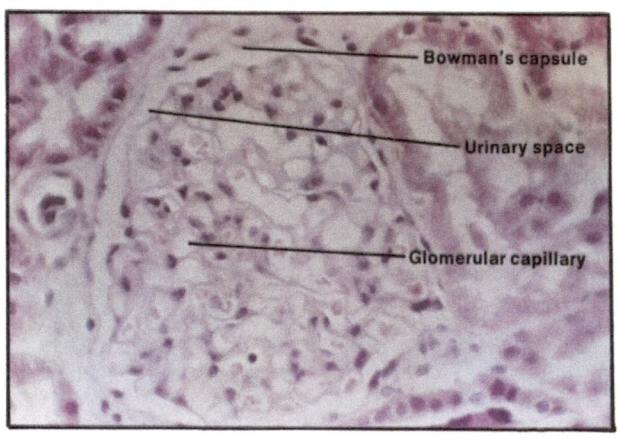

Bowman's capsule

Urinary space

Glomerular capillary

Plate 1. *Normal glomerulus, H and E ×400.*

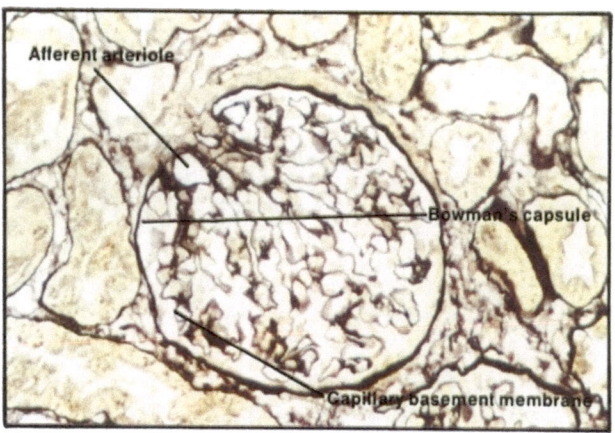

Afferent arteriole

Bowman's capsule

Capillary basement membrane

Plate 2. *Normal glomerulus, silver impregnation ×250.*

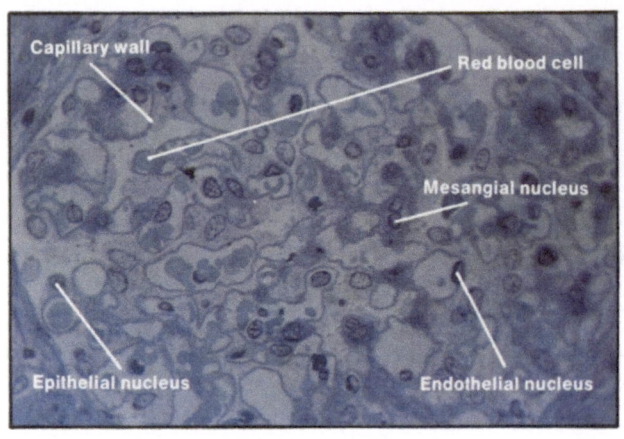

Plate 3. *Normal glomerulus, ultrathin section ×800.*

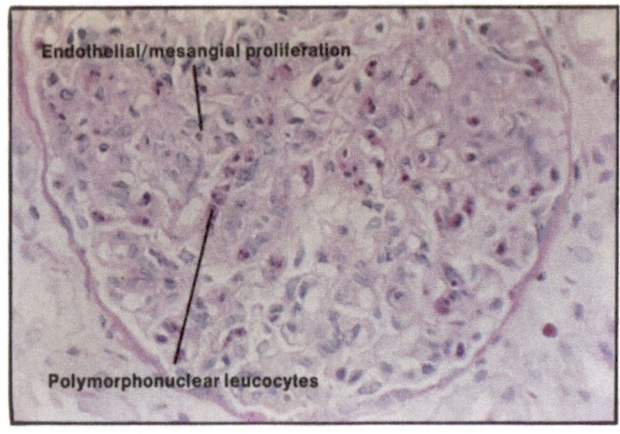

Plate 4. *Diffuse proliferative exudative glomerulonephritis, PAS ×400.*

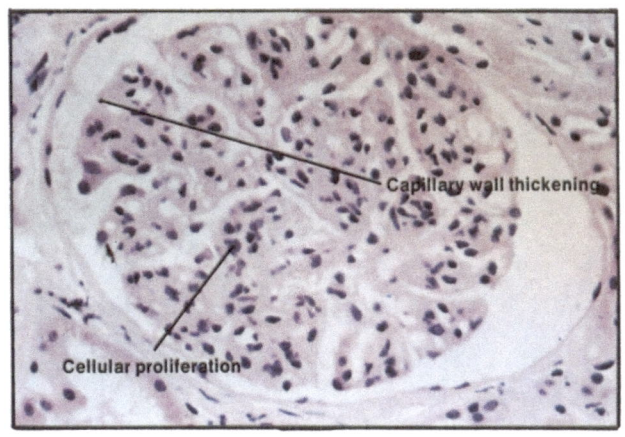

Plate 5. *Mesangiocapillary glomerulonephritis, H and E ×400.*

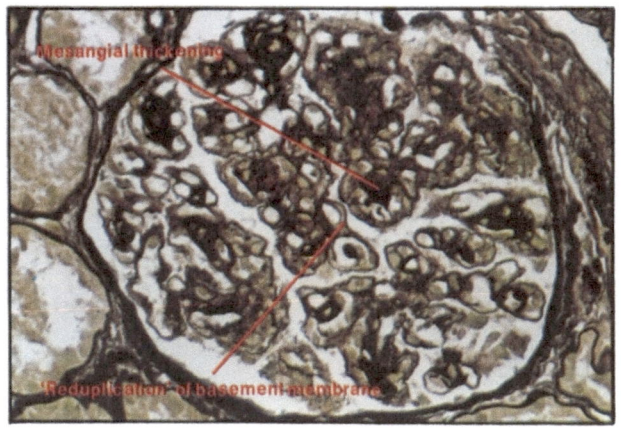

Plate 6. *Mesangiocapillary glomerulonephritis, silver ×400.*

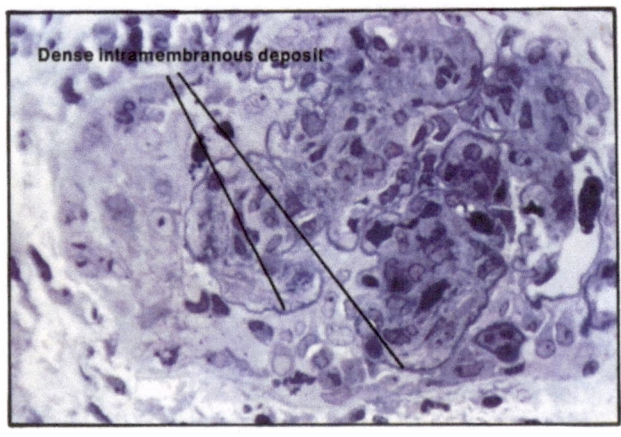

Plate 7. *Mesangiocapillary glomerulonephritis, ultrathin section ×800.*

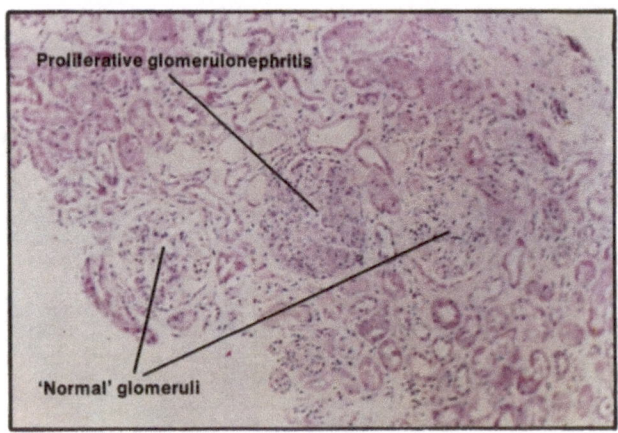

Plate 8. *Focal proliferative glomerulonephritis, H and E ×100.*

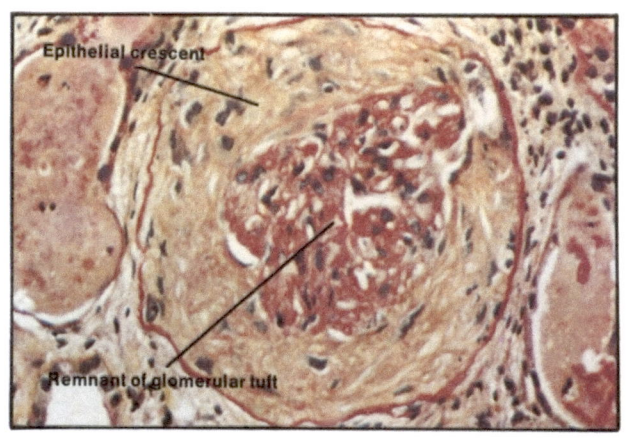

Plate 9. *Proliferative glomerulonephritis with extensive crescents, PAS ×400.*

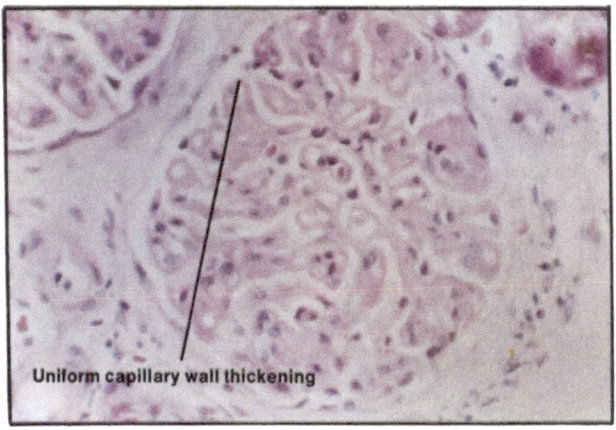

Plate 10. *Membranous nephropathy, H and E ×400.*

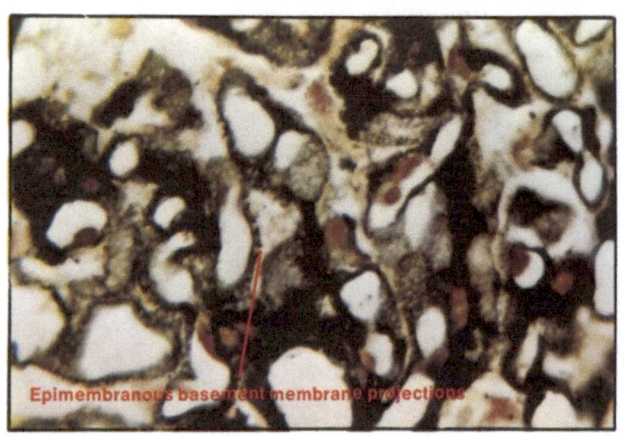

Plate 11. *Membranous nephropathy, silver ×1000.*

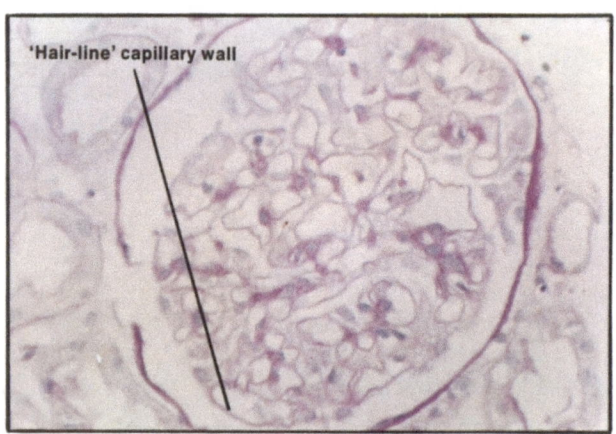

Plate 12. *Minimal change, PAS ×400.*

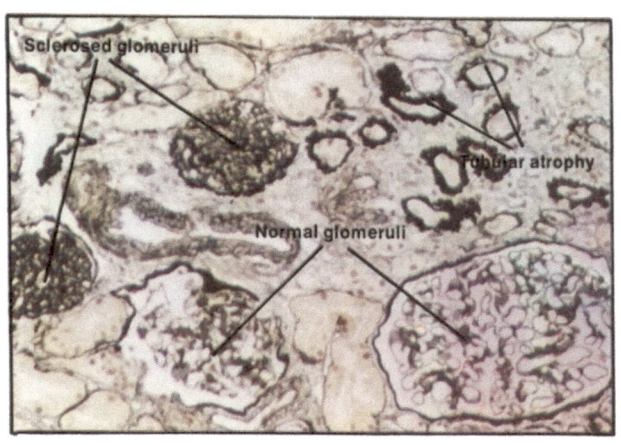

Plate 13. *Focal hyalinosis, silver ×250.*

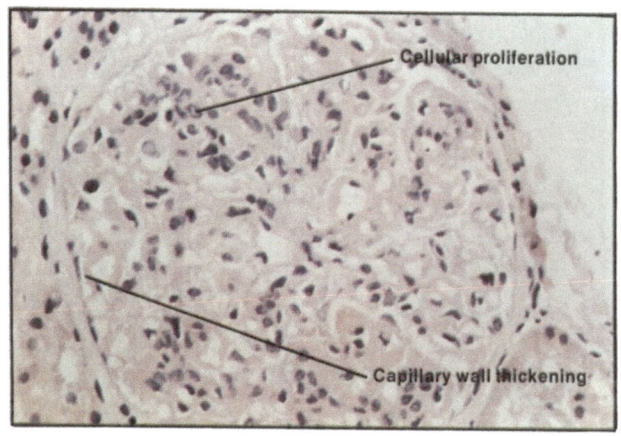

Plate 14. *Systemic lupus erythematosus, H and E ×400.*

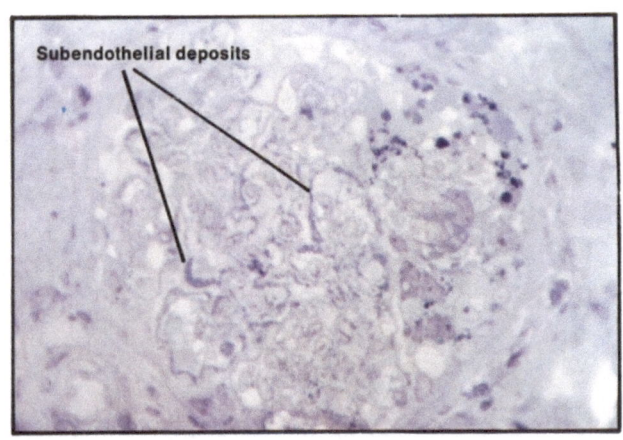

Plate 15. *Systemic lupus erythematosus, ultrathin section ×400.*

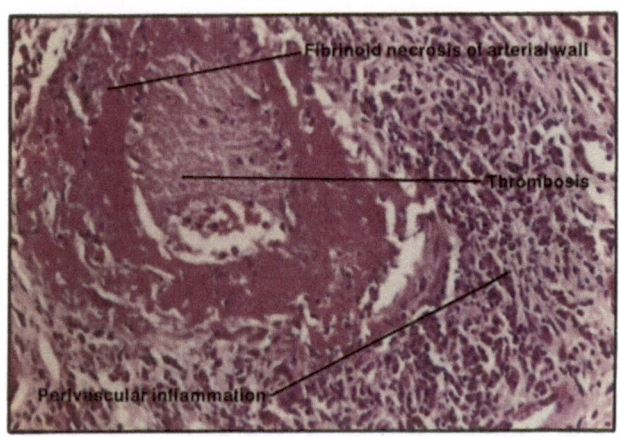

Plate 16. *Polyarteritis nodosa, H and E ×250.*

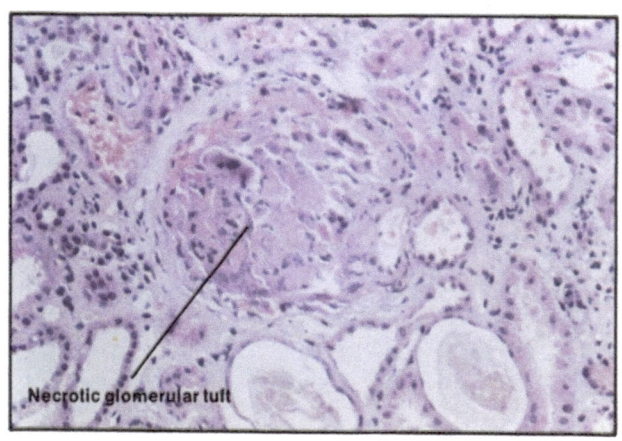

Plate 17. *Polyarteritis nodosa, H and E ×250.*

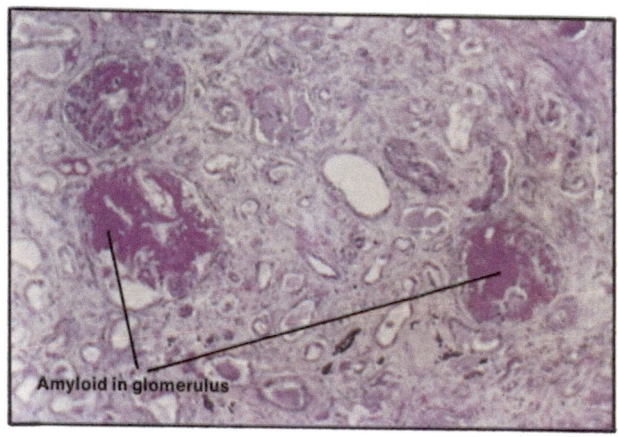

Plate 18. *Amyloidosis, methyl violet ×100.*

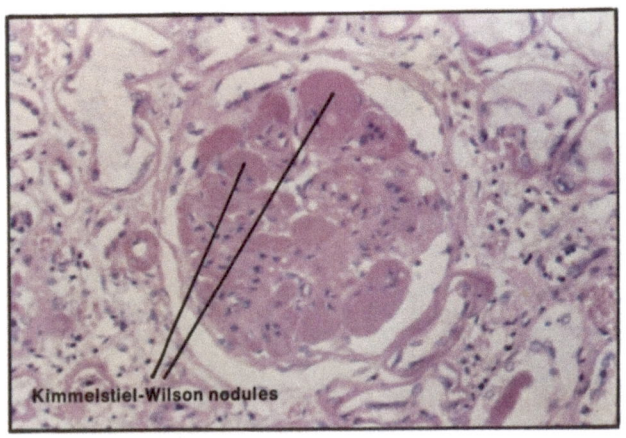

Kimmelstiel-Wilson nodules

Plate 19. *Diabetes, H and E ×250.*

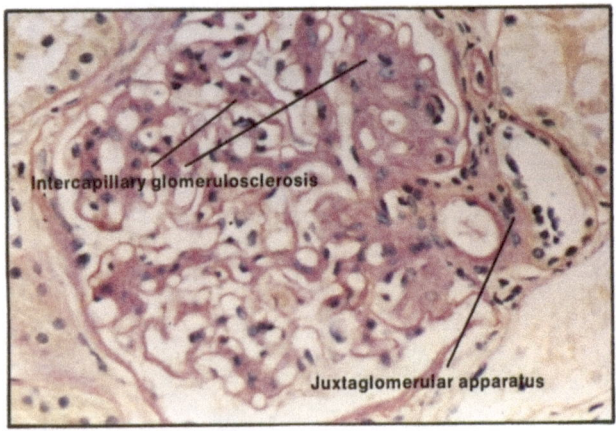

Intercapillary glomerulosclerosis

Juxtaglomerular apparatus

Plate 20. *Diabetes, PAS ×400.*

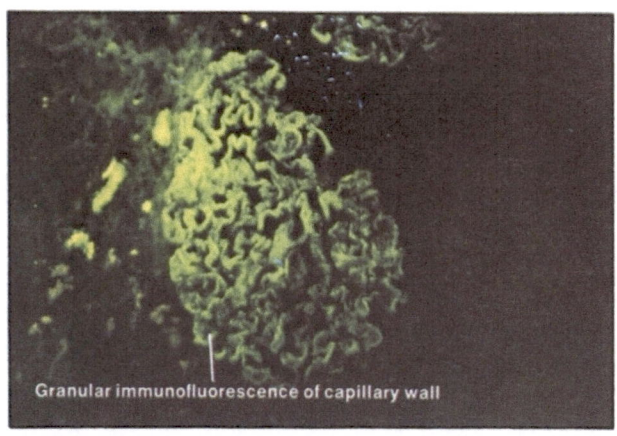

Granular immunofluorescence of capillary wall

Plate 21. *Membranous nephropathy, immunofluorescent microscopy showing granular deposition of IgG.*

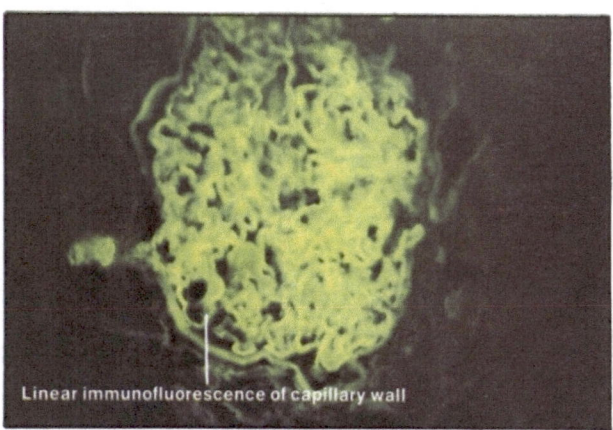

Linear immunofluorescence of capillary wall

Plate 22. *Rapidly progressive glomerulonephritis, immunofluorescent microscopy showing linear deposition of IgG.*

impaired renal function when first seen, and hypertension develops at some stage of the illness in many patients.

A characteristic feature of the disease is that the serum level of C3 (the third component of complement) is reduced at some stage or other in about 80 per cent of the patients. The level may fluctuate, but in the linear deposit variety it is persistently low throughout the course of the illness. This is in contrast to post-streptococcal acute nephritis, in which the C3 concentration is low at the outset but reverts to normal within six weeks.

Although it is not possible to make a definite diagnosis of mesangiocapillary nephritis without renal biopsy, the clinical and laboratory findings can lead to a high order of suspicion. For example, the presence of blood in the urine in a nephrotic, or of more than minimal proteinuria in a patient with recurrent haematuria is highly suggestive. In an acute nephritic illness a persistent reduction in serum C3 is suggestive of this diagnosis.

The prognosis is variable but generally poor. A few patients have shown improvement in renal function, and some die within a few months of presentation, but most run a slowly progressive course, with death from uraemia or hypertension within 10 years of onset.

Focal Proliferative Glomerulonephritis

Focal proliferative glomerulonephritis refers to mesangial or endothelial hypercellularity affecting some of the glomeruli, while the others remain normal (Plate 8). Often there is a segmental distribution as well, in that only parts of individual glomerular tufts are involved. Other changes seen sometimes are areas of necrosis within the tufts, and adhesions between the tuft and Bowman's capsule. Immunofluorescent microscopy, particularly in patients with recurrent haematuria, often shows deposition of IgA in the mesangial regions in all glomeruli, and not just in those with histological abnormalities.

These appearances are most often seen in the clinical setting of a multisystem disease, especially the Henoch–Schönlein syndrome, but they are also found in patients without multisystem disease with the nephrotic syndrome, symptomless proteinuria or isolated haematuria.

The prognosis is uncertain but probably good in most cases. Rarely it progresses to a diffuse glomerulonephritis with corresponding deterioration of renal function.

Proliferative Glomerulonephritis with Extensive Crescent

Crescents are formed by the proliferation of epithelial cells lining Bowman's capsule (Plate 9). Small crescents may be seen in some of the glomeruli in several varieties of glomerulonephritis and even in malignant essential hypertension, but in proliferative glomerulonephritis with extensive crescents they are large and involve most of the glomeruli. These large crescents may fill Bowman's space and in severe cases completely encircle the glomerular tuft. The tufts themselves may show proliferation and in severe cases are compressed, disorganized and even necrotic. They often appear to be strangled by the encircling crescent. In the more chronic cases the cellular crescents become fibrous and the glomerulus undergoes partial or complete sclerosis. Tubular and interstitial damage is correspondingly severe. Immunoglobulin deposition in this condition, particularly in patients with Goodpasture's syndrome, may be in a linear rather than a granular pattern along the basement membrane.

The clinical picture is a rapidly progressive glomerulonephritis, older synonyms for which are sub-acute glomerulonephritis, nephritis with a 'stormy course', rapidly progressive Ellis type I nephritis and acute oliguric glomerulonephritis. The condition may occur at any age, but most commonly affects the middle-aged and elderly. It may present as chronic renal failure, as oliguric acute renal failure of silent onset, or as the nephrotic syndrome. Visible haematuria, heavy proteinuria and red blood cell casts are usually present. The prognosis is extremely poor, end stage renal failure developing within weeks or months of presentation in the majority of cases.

Evidence of a streptococcal aetiology is found in only a few patients. Identical renal histology and a similar clinical course occurs in some cases of Henoch–Schönlein disease, polyarteritis nodosa and Goodpasture's syndrome.

Membranous Nephropathy

Diffuse thickening of the basement membrane involves all capillary loops uniformly and there is no cellular proliferation (Plate 10). However, the H and E stain does not allow the basement membrane to be differentiated from other components of the capillary wall, and other histological techniques are necessary to make a confident diagnosis. With silver staining the basement membrane thickening is seen to be due to a spiky projection of basement membrane material into the epithelial cytoplasm (Plate 11). This is in contrast to mesangiocapillary glomerulonephritis where the basement membrane-like material is deposited internally to the membrane.

Electron microscopy and ultrathin sections show dense deposits on the epithelial side of the basement membrane which correspond to the gaps between the spikes seen in silver-stained preparations. As the disease advances, the basement membranes become thicker, the capillary lumens are obliterated, and ultimately the glomeruli become completely sclerosed. Granular deposition of IgG is the usual finding on immunofluorescent microscopy.

This lesion is rare in childhood. Its common clinical association is the nephrotic syndrome but in the early stages proteinuria may be the only manifestation. The disease is slowly progressive in most cases, renal failure developing gradually and reaching end stage perhaps 10 or 20 years after presentation. However, about 25 per cent of patients remit spontaneously.

Membranous nephropathy is sometimes seen in association with an extrarenal malignancy, especially bronchial carcinoma, and may remit if the tumour is resected. A few cases have also been reported in hepatitis antigen carriers and as a result of penicillamine toxicity.

Minimal Change Disease

Synonyms for minimal change disease are lipoid nephrosis and the idiopathic nephrotic syndrome of childhood. It is a remarkable condition in that, despite their marked permeability to protein, the glomeruli appear virtually normal on light microscopy (Plate

12). Sometimes there is a slight increase in mesangial matrix, and occasionally a few glomeruli are completely sclerosed, but these are really variants of normal renal histology. Electron microscopy is required to demonstrate the only specific abnormality seen, which is fusion of the epithelial cell foot processes (Figure 6). The epithelial cytoplasm appears as a continuous irregular strip applied to the basement membrane instead of as discrete foot processes. The change is reversible and reverts entirely to normal when the disease is in remission, either spontaneous or drug-induced. Droplets of fat in the cytoplasm of the tubules gave the disease its older name of lipoid nephrosis, but these are non-specific and may be seen in other conditions in which there is heavy proteinuria. No immunoglobulins or complement components are shown by immunofluorescent microscopy.

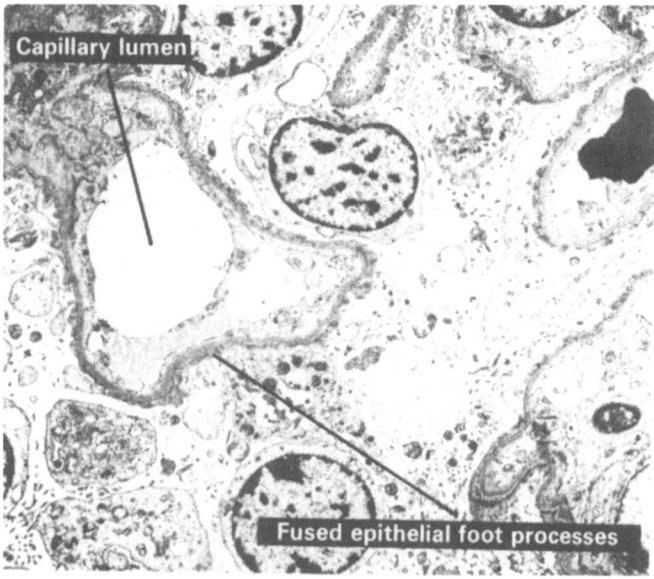

Figure 6. *Minimal change, electron micrograph ×7,000.*

Peak incidence is between the ages of two and ten years, but the condition may occur at any time of life and has been reported in the elderly. At least 90 per cent of childhood nephrotics have the minimal change lesion, while it is the histological appearance in 25 per cent of adults with the nephrotic syndrome. In childhood males are affected three times more commonly than females, whereas in adults the sex incidence is equal.

Minimal change nephrotic syndrome is characterized by heavy proteinuria and usually presents as the nephrotic syndrome. Otherwise there are no features of primary renal dysfunction. There is no hypertension, no haematuria, visible or microscopic, and no cellular casts in the urine. Most importantly, there is no irreversible impairment of renal function, although in some cases there is a reduction in the glomerular filtration rate because of impaired renal blood flow resulting from depletion of circulatory volume. Little structural change occurs in the glomeruli, no matter how long the disease continues, so chronic renal failure does not develop.

Untreated, proteinuria may persist without remission until death occurs from one of the complications of the nephrotic syndrome, but spontaneous remissions often occur, and may last for months or years, or even be permanent. Relapses are often precipitated by incidental infections. Before treatment was available for the kidney lesion or for the complications, the mortality was about 70 per cent. Diuretics, antibiotics, corticosteroids and cytotoxic drugs have now transformed the prognosis to an excellent one.

Focal Hyalinosis

Like focal proliferative glomerulonephritis, this condition (also known as focal glomerulosclerosis) is characterized by involvement of some of the glomeruli, while the others remain normal. It differs in that there is no excess of cells, merely a hyaline thickening of mesangial regions and capillary loops (Plate 13), initially with a segmental distribution within the glomerulus. As hyalinization increases, the whole glomerulus becomes obliterated. Gradually more glomeruli are involved and ultimately all of them, but the lesion remains focal until the late stages of the disease. The glomerulosclerosis is accompanied by a patchy tubular atrophy. IgM and C3 in a granular pattern are seen in the histologically abnormal glomeruli, but not in the others.

The earliest glomeruli to be involved are those in the deepest (or juxtamedullary) regions of the cortex. Because of the sampling error of renal biopsy, all the glomeruli obtained may be normal, and the condition is easily confused with minimal change.

Focal hyalinosis mainly affects children, and usually presents as the nephrotic syndrome. Clinically it differs from the minimal change nephrotic syndrome by the presence, usually, of microscopic haematuria and the fact that renal function becomes progressively impaired. The rate of progress is variable but is usually slow, and it may be five or ten years before end stage renal failure develops. Another important difference from the minimal change lesion is that there is no response to corticosteroids. It may well be that the small proportion of minimal change patients who reportedly failed to respond to steroids in fact had focal hyalinosis.

Unclassified Glomerular Lesions

Even the most experienced kidney pathologist is unable to fit many biopsies into one of the above categories, particularly when the disease is advanced. In these cases it is much better to leave the diagnosis open than to make an assumption which may very well be wrong.

Multisystem Disease

The glomeruli are involved by a disease process which affects other parts of the body as well. With the exception of diabetes, amyloid and lupus erythematosus, the renal lesion is rarely specific, and the pathologist is unable to distinguish the appearances from those of the various types of primary glomerulonephritis.

Systemic Lupus Erythematosus (SLE)

A wide variety of renal lesions may be seen in SLE (Plate 14), usually some combination of cellular proliferation and necrosis, thickening of the capillary wall, epithelial crescents and glomerular hyalinization. Often only localized areas of the tuft are involved by proliferation and necrosis, and there may be adhesions to Bowman's capsule at these sites. In addition the capillary wall thickening is often local, affecting some capillary loops and not others, although occasionally there is diffuse thickening, giving an appearance similar to membranous nephropathy. Electron microscopy shows that there is true thickening of the basement membrane itself, and subendothelial deposition of electron-dense material often contributes to the capillary wall thickening. These deposits may also be seen by light microscopy in ultrathin sections (Plate 15). A common finding is the filling of capillary loops by fibrinoid material to form so-called hyaline thrombi.

A specific feature, but one which is uncommonly observed, is the presence of haematoxyphil bodies. These are ill-defined structures in the glomerular tuft, smaller than nuclei, and staining lilac or purple with H and E. They consist of damaged nuclei and correspond to the inclusion bodies of LE cells.

Immunofluorescent staining reveals granular deposition of IgG in all cases, of C3, Clq and C4 in most, and of other immunoglobulins and fibrinogen in some.

The distribution of the glomerular lesion has an important bearing on the outcome. When there is a focal distribution, prognosis is much better than when there is a diffuse glomerulonephritis. It is unusual for the focal variety to progress to the diffuse one. In the progressive cases glomeruli become increasingly hyalinized and there is corresponding tubular and interstitial damage. There are usually no remarkable blood vessel changes, although occasionally a necrotizing arteritis is seen.

Clinically about 50 per cent of patients with SLE have evidence of renal involvement, though at autopsy the proportion is much higher. Many patients have proteinuria of only a small degree and this corresponds to the minor histological lesions. Microscopic haematuria is common as well. The nephrotic syndrome or impaired renal function are more serious manifestations. In these patients the disease is usually slowly progressive, although spontaneous remissions may occur.

Polyarteritis Nodosa

Most patients with polyarteritis nodosa have renal involvement. This is of two main types, which may occur separately or together. In the first type there is segmental necrosis and fibrinoid change in the walls of medium and small arteries with a surrounding acute inflammation and intraluminal thrombosis (Plate 16). Ischaemia distal to the occluded vessels results in infarcts of varying size. Healing occurs by organization of the thrombus and fibrosis of the vessel wall. In the second type the glomerular capillaries are mainly involved. There is a proliferative glomerulonephritis, which is non-specific, and local areas of necrosis and fibrinoid change in the tuft are common (Plate 17).

In most cases immunofluorescent microscopy shows no immunoglobulin or complement deposits. The clinical features depend on the size of vessel damaged. In the larger vessel form of the disease, the symptoms are those of renal infarctions with episodes of loin pain and haematuria, and there is a high incidence of hypertension, which is sometimes malignant. Renal function remains well preserved however. The small vessel or glomerular disease is less common and is characterized by proteinuria, haematuria, and impairment of renal function, which is often rapidly progressive with end stage renal failure developing within a few weeks of onset. In other patients the downhill course is less rapid.

Henoch–Schönlein Syndrome

The commonest picture of renal involvement in Henoch–Schönlein syndrome is a focal proliferative glomerulonephritis (Plate 8), often with local areas of necrosis in the glomeruli. A few patients have a diffuse glomerulonephritis with proliferation in all the glomeruli and sometimes extensive epithelial crescents (Plate 9). Some patients with clinical manifestations of renal disease have only minimal lesions on kidney biopsy.

The peak incidence is between the ages of two and five years, and it is less common in adults. The reported frequency of renal involvement in Henoch–Schönlein disease varies widely and has been up to 50 per cent in some series. The onset usually occurs within a few weeks of the systemic symptoms, and many of the patients have only minor urinary abnormalities, such as microscopic haematuria and a small degree of proteinuria. It may present as an acute nephritis-like illness with macroscopic haematuria and proteinuria, or there may be a nephrotic syndrome. In general, the prognosis is good; two thirds of patients recover completely and most of the remainder are left with urinary abnormalities but little or no impairment of renal function. However, a few patients, those with diffuse disease and large crescents, run a rapidly progressive course to develop end stage renal failure within a few months. A higher proportion of adults than of children develops this severe variety of the disease.

Goodpasture's Syndrome

The pathological and clinical features of the renal lesion in Goodpasture's syndrome are similar to those of rapidly progressive glomerulonephritis. Only the pulmonary haemorrhage distinguishes Goodpasture's syndrome. There is extensive glomerular destruction by proliferation, necrosis and crescents.

Immunofluorescent microscopy characteristically shows IgG and C3 deposited along the basement membrane in a *linear* fashion.

The disease mostly affects young adult males and usually presents with haemoptysis followed by anaemia and dyspnoea. The renal manifestations start with macroscopic haematuria and then renal impairment develops, usually leading to death within a few weeks or months. The prognosis is very poor, but there is a handful of long-term survivors.

Renal Amyloidosis

Classically, renal involvement was said to occur in amyloid secondary to other diseases, such as tuberculosis, chronic suppuration, rheumatoid arthritis and multiple myeloma, but in the UK it has an equal incidence in the so-called primary disease. In countries with a high incidence of predisposing causes, such as tuberculosis or familial Mediterranean fever, amyloidosis is much more common.

With H and E staining amyloid is seen as irregular, hyaline, eosinophilic, extracellular material. It is prominent in the glomeruli, initially in the mesangial regions, and later in the capillary wall as well. It encroaches on the lumina and eventually may completely obliterate the glomeruli. Deposits are also found in the basement membrane of the tubules, in vessel walls and in the interstitium.

Early amyloid may be difficult to diagnose with routine histological methods and its staining characteristics vary, so special stains are required. Methyl violet stains amyloid tissue red (Plate 18), Congo Red stains it pink and causes birefringence with polarization microscopy, and thioflavine T produces fluorescence under ultraviolet light. No single method is uniformly successful, so several should be used. Electron microscopy shows a characteristic fibrillary structure, and is the most reliable method of diagnosis.

Using sensitive techniques a high incidence of myeloma-type protein is found in the serum or the urine of patients with the primary disease and there is evidence that the amyloid fibrils are derived from light chain fragments. On the other hand, the fibrils of secondary amyloidosis can be formed from many polypeptides resulting from tissue destruction by a variety of pathological processes.

Renal amyloidosis is not a rare condition, even in patients with no predisposing disease; an incidence as high as 10 per cent has been found in one series of unselected adult nephrotics (Sharpstone et al. 1969). The most consistent clinical feature is proteinuria, which is often heavy enough to produce the nephrotic syndrome. Renal insufficiency is mild in many cases at the time of diagnosis, and the histological abnormality often appears disproportionately severe in comparison with the impairment of function. Hypertension may occur with advanced disease. The condition progresses slowly to terminal renal failure unless the primary cause can be treated successfully, in which case it usually remains stationary rather than disappearing. An occasional but important complication is renal vein thrombosis.

Diabetic Nephropathy

Four main glomerular abnormalities occur, either singly or in combination, in diabetic nephropathy. The first, only seen in a few cases, is the only one specific for diabetes. This is the nodular lesion of Kimmelstiel and Wilson, which comprises a rounded, homogeneous, eosinophilic, PAS-positive lesion in the centre of a lobule near the periphery of the tuft (Plate 19). When more than one lesion is present in a single glomerulus they usually differ in size. The second type, diffuse intercapillary glomerulosclerosis (Plate 20), is more common than the Kimmelstiel–Wilson lesion. It consists of an increase in eosinophilic PAS-positive material in the mesangium, giving an appearance similar to that seen in the more sclerotic varieties of mesangial proliferative glomerulo-nephritis. There is usually irregular thickening of the capillary walls as well. The third lesion is the 'fibrin cap', which is an eosinophilic, crescentic structure applied to a capillary loop, usually at the periphery of a lobule. The fourth, the 'capsular drop', is a small eosinophilic nodule on the inner surface of Bowman's capsule.

Electron microscopy shows that there is thickening of the capillary basement membrane, and that the nodular and the intercapillary deposits are composed of basement membrane-like material originating in the mesangium.

The vascular changes in the diabetic kidney are very important. Qualitatively they are similar to those which occur in ageing and in benign hypertension, but their severity is out of proportion to the patient's age and blood pressure. Hyaline thickening of arteriolar walls is particularly prominent.

As the diabetic lesion progresses, capillary lumina are reduced, collagen is laid down internal to Bowman's capsule, the tuft shrinks, and eventually the glomerulus becomes completely hyalinized. Tubules become atrophic and the interstitium fibrosed. The glomerular lesions and the arteriosclerosis both contribute to this progressive destruction of the kidney.

Foci of acute and chronic inflammatory cells are often found in the interstitium and in the past have been interpreted as indicating chronic pyelonephritis. But this inflammation is not necessarily due to bacterial infection, and even though diabetics are predisposed to acute urinary infection it is doubtful that true chronic pyelonephritis plays much part in diabetic kidney damage. Another important renal complication is papillary necrosis, which is much more frequent in diabetics than in the general population.

About two thirds of diabetics have renal lesions demonstrable by light microscopy and nearly all have abnormalities on electron microscopy. The typical nodules are seen in about one fifth. The renal involvement tends to be more severe in patients who develop diabetes at an early age and to increase with the duration of the disease. It is probably aggravated by poor control of the diabetes. Most patients with significant renal involvement have retinopathy as well.

The commonest clinical manifestation is proteinuria alone. This is only infrequently heavy enough to produce the nephrotic syndrome. The glomerulosclerosis progresses slowly and renal function becomes insidiously impaired. The correlation between histological changes and renal function is poor, however, and the rate of deterioration varies widely from patient to patient. Some patients with impaired renal function survive for many years with no further deterioration. Heavy proteinuria, however, is an ominous sign and end stage renal failure usually ensues within a few years. Hypertension is common, even when renal function is well preserved.

5. Aetiology and Pathogenesis

The list of common glomerular diseases in which the causative agent is known is short:

1. Post-streptococcal glomerulonephritis.
2. Malarial nephrosis.

In these conditions, and a few less common ones, there is good evidence that the exogenous agent sets off a chain of immunological reactions which ultimately cause the kidney damage. In many other types of nephritis immunological mechanisms also seem to play a part in the pathogenesis, but the triggering agent is unknown. Humoral antibodies rather than cell-mediated immunological reactions seem to be of prime importance in glomerular disease. The evidence comes both from experimental and clinical sources.

Experimental Nephritis

Serum Sickness Nephritis

Rabbits injected with albumin from another species of mammal, such as the cow, develop an acute nephritis, as well as other manifestations of serum sickness. Characteristically there is a latent interval of seven to nine days between the injection and the onset of the illness.

Immunoglobulins and components of complement are demonstrable as granular deposits on the basement membrane by immunofluorescent staining (Plate 21). Here the antigen (bovine albumin) combines with rabbit immunoglobulin in the circulation to form antigen–antibody complexes. In conditions of slight antigen excess these complexes are small enough to avoid being taken up by the reticuloendothelial system and they circulate in the bloodstream as soluble complexes. They are, however, too large to be filtered through the glomerular basement membrane, so they lodge there and incite a local inflammatory reaction by mechanisms described below (Figure 7).

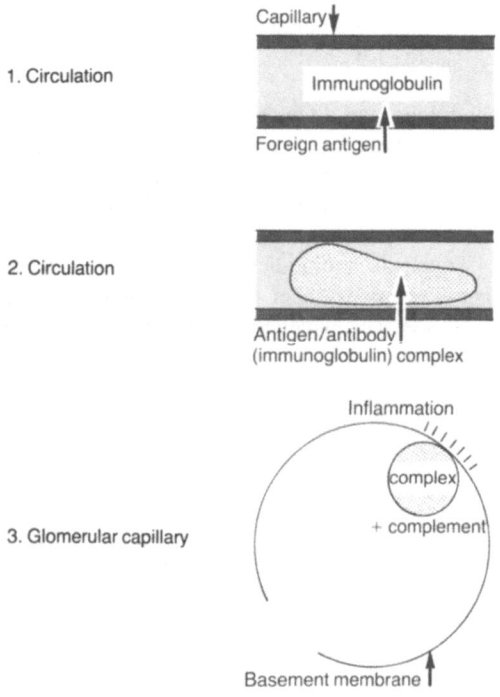

Figure 7. *Schema of experimental serum sickness nephritis.*

Repeated Injections of Antigen

If the injections of foreign albumin are repeated at carefully chosen intervals and doses, it is possible to produce chronic progressive glomerular damage in the rabbit.

Virus-induced Nephritis

In some animals certain chronic virus infections, such as lymphocytic choriomeningitis virus in mice, can produce a glomerulonephritis, and there is evidence that the damage is immunologically mediated.

Autoimmune Nephritis

All members of a particular species of hybrid mouse (NZB/NZW) spontaneously develop a progressive nephritis together with other manifestations of an SLE-like illness. The antigen in the circulating complexes is the animal's own DNA, suggesting a true autoimmune pathogenesis. It remains possible, however, that the DNA is liberated by an exogenous agent, such as a virus, to which that particular species of mouse is susceptible.

Nephrotoxic Serum Nephritis

It is possible to produce nephritis in animals by a mechanism entirely different to those described above. A suspension of kidney tissue from an animal of one species is injected into one of another species. Serum from the second animal causes nephritis when injected into a member of the original species (Figure 8). By using isolated basement membrane material rather than whole kidney for the immunization it can be shown that it is the basement membrane itself which acts as the antigen. Thus antibody specifically directed against glomerular basement membrane, rather than antigen–antibody complexes, causes the damage here. Such antiglomerular basement membrane antibodies are demonstrated by immunofluorescent microscopy as continuous or linear deposits along the basement membrane (Plate 22).

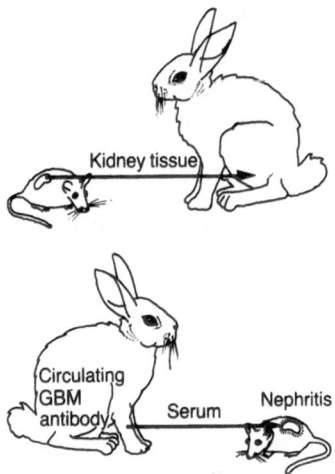

Figure 8. *Schema of experimental nephrotoxic (antiglomerular basement membrane) nephritis.*

Human Glomerulonephritis

Striking counterparts to the animal experiments suggest that some human types of glomerulonephritis may be immunologically mediated, although the evidence is not conclusive.

Post-streptococcal Glomerulonephritis

The latent period between infection with the streptococcus and the onset of nephritis resembles that between the injection and the onset of serum sickness nephritis. Immunofluorescence shows basement membrane deposits of IgG in the granular distribution characteristic of immune complex disease. Electron microscopy during the acute phase shows subepithelial humps (Figure 5), which are thought to be the immune complexes themselves. Some component of the streptococcus is presumed to be the antigen, but specific streptococcal material has not yet been identified in the basement membrane deposits.

Malarial Nephrosis

Malarial nephrosis has all the hallmarks of an antigen–antibody complex disease, and there are very good epidemiological grounds for incriminating the parasite of quartan malaria as the inciting agent. Further, malarial antigen has been demonstrated in the glomeruli.

Systemic Lupus Erythematosus

IgG is found regularly and other immunoglobulins less frequently in the glomeruli in lupus nephritis. Their distribution is granular and there is good evidence that endogenous DNA is the antigen in the complexes.

Membranous Nephropathy

The presence of immunoglobulins in a granular pattern and electron-dense deposits along the basement membrane indicates immune complex disease. In most patients the nature of the antigen is unknown, but when the condition occurs in association with malignancy elsewhere in the body, in hepatitis carriers, and as the result of penicillamine, gold or mercury toxicity, the antigens responsible are tumour tissue, hepatitis antigens and the toxin, respectively.

Other Varieties of Chronic Glomerulonephritis

Granular deposition of immunoglobulins occurs in other varieties of proliferative glomerulonephritis, and in focal hyalinosis, suggesting that these are immune-complex disorders, but the nature of the antigen in these cases is unknown. By analogy with the animal diseases it is tempting to speculate that so far undetected 'slow' viruses may be responsible in some cases.

Goodpasture's Syndrome

In Goodpasture's syndrome and in some other patients with rapidly progressive glomerulonephritis immunoglobulins are found in a linear distribution on the basement membrane (Plate 22). This suggests that antiglomerular basement membrane antibodies are responsible, and such antibodies have been identified in the circulation and urine of these patients. Nevertheless, it remains possible that the stimulus to the formation of antibodies is a non-immunological one.

It seems that kidney rather than lung basement membrane antigen is responsible for the continued production of antibody since, in a number of patients, bilateral nephrectomy has resulted in regression of the lung lesion.

Minimal Change Lesion

Here there is very little evidence of an immunological or any other pathogenesis. Although a few subjects with hay fever have exacerbations of the nephrotic syndrome during the pollen season and IgE is said to have been demonstrated in the glomeruli, the place of reaginic antibody has not been established in most of the patients investigated.

Mediation of Injury

Complement

Much of the damage caused by the immune complexes trapped in the glomeruli is mediated by the local activation of complement. The first (C1) of the nine components of complement binds to antigen–antibody complexes and is converted to a proteolytic enzyme which acts on the next two components (C2 and C4) resulting in the formation of another enzyme which activates C3. The subsequent components in the complement chain are then activated sequentially in a similar manner (Figure 9). The terminal components of complement have numerous effects, including attraction of polymorphonuclear leucocytes, release of histamine and enzymes, platelet aggregation and cell destruction, which result in an inflammatory reaction and increased capillary permeability. The complement system may also be activated by non-immunological mechanisms via an alternative pathway to the classical one, in which the gamma globulin properdin acts at the level of C3, so that the earlier components (C1, C2 and C4) are not involved.

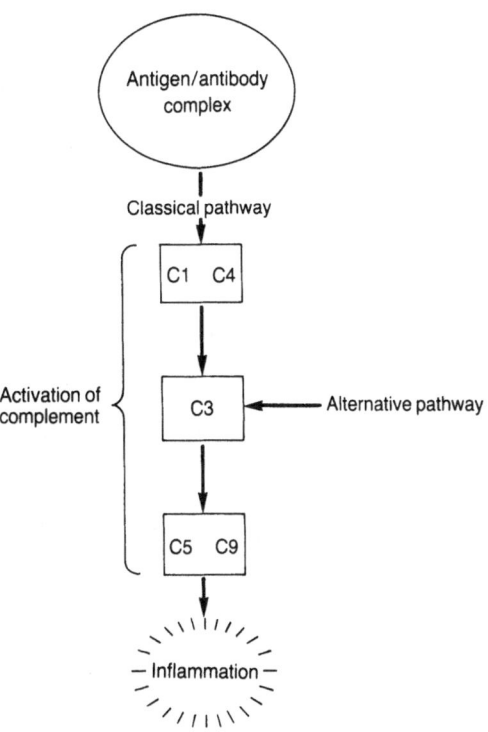

Figure 9. *Schema of activation of complement.*

Complement in Human Nephritis

The participation of the complement system in human nephritis is suggested by the presence of C3 along the basement membrane in many varieties of glomerulonephritis. In some the serum level of C3 is reduced as well.

In post-streptococcal glomerulonephritis the serum C3 is low during the acute phase of the illness but the level of C4 is normal, suggesting activation of the complement system by the alternative pathway. In lupus nephritis C4 as well as C3 is reduced during the active phases, indicating activation of the system by the classic pathway. In mesangiocapillary glomerulonephritis the C3 (but not C4) is persistently low in most cases. The reduction persists after nephrectomy in these patients, so utilization in the kidney cannot be the cause. There is, however, a factor (C3 nephritic factor) in the serum of patients with mesangiocapillary glomerulonephritis which activates C3 and this is probably the cause of the persistent hypocomplementaemia.

Coagulation

Both the terminal components of complement and immune complexes themselves cause platelet aggregation and activation of the coagulation mechanism. In some glomerular diseases, especially severe proliferative glomerulonephritis with crescents, deposits of fibrin are often observed in the glomeruli by conventional microscopy. In many other cases fibrinogen can be identified along the basement membrane by immunofluorescence. In addition, degradation products of fibrin are often found in the urine of patients with active glomerular disease and it may be that the fibrin is one of the factors causing glomerular damage by obliterating capillaries and by provoking an inflammatory reaction.

Repair

Acute inflammation of the glomeruli does not necessarily destroy the glomeruli, as exemplified by the usual complete recovery after the florid inflammatory reaction in post-streptococcal acute glomerulonephritis. In chronic glomerulonephritis with serious impairment of kidney function, however, it is usual to see considerable sclerosis of the glomeruli. This scarring represents attempts at repair of repeated or continued insults, and it is this which is responsible for the permanent damage.

6. Investigations and Their Interpretation

Laboratory investigations required in patients with glomerular disease are listed in Table 3. Technical details are outside the scope of this book, but some practical points in their performance and interpretation are discussed.

Table 3. Investigations in glomerular disease.

Urine	
'Stix' tests	Protein
	Blood
Microscopy	RBCs
	WBCs
	Casts
Protein	24-hour excretion
Protein selectivity	
Renal function	
Blood urea	
Plasma creatinine	
Creatinine clearance	
Glomerular filtration rate	
Serum	
Albumin	
Immunoglobulins	
Complement components	
Antinuclear factor	
Intravenous Urogram (IVU)	
Biopsy	

Urine

'Stix' Tests

The 'Stix' tests for blood and albumin in urine are sensitive and valuable tests provided the makers' instructions are followed scrupulously, and the method's limitations borne in mind. For routine purposes they have supplanted the older semiquantitative methods.

'Haemastix' is very sensitive to free haemoglobin but less so to intact red cells. Microscopy is needed to exclude trace amounts of blood, and to be sure that haematuria is present rather than haemoglobinuria. Haemoglobinuria may, of course, occur in various haemolytic disorders and is not necessarily an indication of disease of the urinary tract.

'Albustix' is very sensitive to albumin and it must be remembered that a trace result (0.05 to 0.2 g/l) encompasses the range of physiological protein excretion and does not necessarily indicate pathological proteinuria.

Many different proteins may appear in the urine in renal disease, but Albustix is much more sensitive to albumin than the others. This does not detract from the value of the test since pathological proteinuria will virtually always include the lower molecular weight proteins of which albumin is one. An exception is Bence-Jones proteinuria, which may occur in the absence of albuminuria, but it must be rare to diagnose myeloma by routine urine testing alone.

The simplicity of Albustix makes it suitable for use by patients themselves, for example by those with a relapsing nephrotic syndrome.

Proteinuria has many causes other than renal disease and, conversely, the absence of proteinuria does not exclude disease of the urinary tract. Occasionally, it may even be absent in glomerular disease.

Urine Microscopy

A heavy deposit may be examined in unspun urine, but a lighter one needs centrifugation. This should be for no more than five minutes, otherwise casts may be destroyed. Important practical points to remember during the examination of the unstained deposit are to stop down the diaphragm so that the field is not too bright, and to be sure to focus in the correct plane. Much time and energy has been expended by novices in the inspection of dust particles on the surface of the cover slip! It is helpful to focus on areas adjacent to the edge of the cover slip first, since cells often congregate there. The identification of components of the sediment requires practice under skilled supervision.

More than two red blood cells per high power field is abnormal. In the absence of vaginal bleeding, including menstruation, it indicates disease of the urinary tract but not necessarily of the renal parenchyma.

Up to five white blood cells per high power field may be normal and an excess indicates an inflammatory lesion of the urinary tract. It is not diagnostic of pyelonephritis since pyuria may be found in patients with glomerulonephritis and other urinary tract disorders.

The finding of red cell or granular casts in the urine is important since these originate in the tubules and must indicate renal parenchymal disease. When there is haematuria the presence of accompanying red cell casts is valuable in identifying the kidney as the site of the bleeding. Hyaline casts have no pathological significance.

Quantitative Urine Protein

The concentration of protein in the urine varies during a 24-hour period and the only accurate method of quantitating the rate of protein excretion is to measure the total 24-hour output. This will depend on an accurate 24-hour urine collection and precise instructions, written as well as oral, must be given to the patient. In particular it should be emphasized that he must discard the first specimen at the beginning of the 24-hour period and should empty his bladder fully into the container at the end of the 24 hours.

Protein excretion of more than 2 g/24 hr usually indicates glomerular disease, but lesser amounts by no means exclude it. Serial measurements are useful in following the patient's progress and response to treatment, but the values must be interpreted in conjunction with measurements of renal function. As renal function deteriorates proteinuria tends to diminish since fewer glomeruli are available for filtration.

Urine Protein Excretion Selectivity

In the nephrotic syndrome a knowledge of the pattern of excretion of proteins of different molecular weights gives some indication of the severity of the glomerular disease. In serious diseases the glomeruli tend to be permeable to proteins of larger molecular weight than in some less serious disorders.

Quantitation of a large number of proteins is tedious and a relatively simple test is to measure the concentration of two proteins in plasma and urine by an immunodiffusion method. The two chosen, transferrin and IgG, represent low and high molecular weights, respectively. The relationship between the ratios of their urine/plasma concentrations gives an index of the relative permeability of the glomeruli to them.

The clearance of IgG is expressed as a proportion of the clearance of transferrin:

$$\frac{(UV/P) \; IgG}{(UV/P) \; transferrin}$$

where
U is the urine concentration
P the plasma concentration
V the urine volume.

Since both proteins are measured in the same samples, the urine volumes can be ignored.

The figure derived is known as the 'selectivity index'. A value greater than 0.20 indicates that a large amount of IgG is being excreted in relation to transferrin, and the proteinuria is said to be poorly selective. A selectivity index of less than 0.20 indicates selective proteinuria, that is predominantly low molecular weight proteins are getting through. In practice the main value of the test is an aid to the diagnosis of the minimal change nephrotic syndrome, in which proteinuria is usually highly selective.

Renal Function

Blood Urea and Creatinine

The most important guide to the severity of a renal lesion is a measurement of glomerular filtration rate (GFR), which directly reflects the number of functioning nephrons remaining. Unfortunately, the blood urea concentration is not such a measure. First, it may not rise at all until the GFR has fallen to one third or less of normal; and second, it is influenced by factors other than renal function, i.e. the quantity of protein ingested and the rate of endogenous protein breakdown. Thus the blood urea may be elevated with normal renal function if a very high protein diet is eaten or if the patient has severe sepsis or tissue damage. Conversely, the blood urea may be normal with a GFR as low as one fifth of normal if the protein intake is kept very low. Nevertheless, if these limitations are remembered, serial measurement of blood urea remains a useful clinical guide. Since the serum creatinine concentration is not influenced by protein intake or catabolism, it is more reliable.

Glomerular Filtration Rate

GFR is measured by determining the clearance by the urine of a substance in the plasma which is excreted by glomerular filtration alone and is not secreted or reabsorbed by the tubules. This substance must circulate freely in the extracellular fluid and not be degraded or excreted by non-renal routes. Such a substance is inulin, which is used as a standard of reference for all other methods. Since inulin is not normally present in the body it must be given intravenously to produce an appropriate plasma concentration, and then it is infused intravenously at a rate calculated to maintain the serum concentration at that level, while urine collections are made at timed intervals. The clearance is calculated from the formula

$$\frac{UV}{P}$$

where
U is the urine concentration of inulin
P the plasma concentration of inulin in the same units
V the rate of urine excretion in ml/min.

The normal GFR is about 120 ml/min. It tends to be higher in men than women and should be corrected to a body surface area of 1.73 m^2 for accuracy, especially in children.

However, measurement of inulin clearance is not practicable for clinical use. An intravenous infusion must be given and urine collections very accurately timed, since the collection periods are necessarily short. There may be difficulty in complete bladder emptying during these short periods. Further, the chemical assay of inulin is tedious.

For these reasons in clinical practice the clearance of creatinine is usually used to measure GFR. Since creatinine is normally present in the plasma, no infusion is needed. Its level is reasonably constant so collection periods can be prolonged to 24 hours, and the accuracy of urine collection becomes less crucial. Unfortunately the chemical assay of creatinine is not entirely specific and there is some degree of tubular secretion. However, as long as it is remembered that creatinine clearance does not measure GFR precisely, it is a very useful clinical test. The range of normal is greater than that of inulin clearance and less attention should be paid to small variations.

A recent advance in the clinical assessment of GFR is the use of isotopically labelled exogenous markers of glomerular filtration. One such is the chelating agent, EDTA, labelled with the isotope, chromium 51 (^{51}Cr EDTA). This has the advantage over inulin in that it is measured simply by counting its radioactivity. A further refinement is to dispense with urine collections by giving a single intravenous injection of the material and calculating the GFR from the rate of fall of its plasma concentration. This 'single shot' method is very easy to carry out, involving only one injection and two or three blood samples; but it is unreliable in the presence of oedema, since equilibration of the marker in the extracellular fluid is prolonged.

Serum

Serum Proteins

The plasma globulin pattern may give a clue to the presence of a multisystem disease, such as myeloma or SLE, while the serum albumin is important to assess the consequence of proteinuria. However heavy the proteinuria, oedema is unlikely until the serum albumin concentration is less than 30 g/l and often it is much lower. The serum albumin is not, however, a reliable guide to the progress of the kidney lesion since it is affected by the rate of albumin synthesis as well as by its excretion. Elderly patients tend to synthesize albumin less well than younger ones, so they become oedematous with smaller degrees of protein excretion. Also younger patients often tolerate lower levels of serum albumin without developing oedema.

Serum Complement and Complement Components

There are many methods of measuring serum complement and its numerous components. For clinical purposes at present a measurement of the third component, C3, and sometimes Clq and C4, suffices. These may be carried out by a simple immuno-diffusion technique.

A persistent depression of C3 is an aid to the differentiation of mesangiocapillary glomerulonephritis from other types, since it is persistently low in most patients with this condition. Depression of Clq and C4 as well as C3 may assist in the diagnosis of lupus nephritis.

Antinuclear Factor and Anti-DNA Antibody

Antinuclear factor and anti-DNA antibody should be tested for as a routine in glomerulonephritis of uncertain aetiology, since lupus nephritis may present without any other clinical features of SLE, and renal biopsy may be non-specific. Anti-DNA antibody in the serum is more specific for SLE than antinuclear factor. Its presence in high titre generally indicates active (particularly renal) disease and a rising titre may herald the onset of clinical activity.

For these reasons assay of anti-DNA antibody is more valuable than antinuclear factor in the assessment of patients with renal lupus.

Intravenous Urogram

The value of the intravenous urogram (IVU) has been enhanced in recent years by the recognition that a useful picture can be obtained even in patients with severely depressed renal function if a high enough dose (2 ml/kg body weight) of the contrast medium is used. With a sufficiently large dose, preliminary dehydration of the patient, which is dangerous in uraemia, is unnecessary. Its particular uses in nephrology are as follows:

1. To exclude lesions of the lower urinary tract.

2. To diagnose structural lesions of the kidney, such as polycystic disease and chronic pyelonephritis.

3. To demonstrate the size of the kidneys; small kidneys indicate severe irreversible damage.

4. To locate the kidneys for biopsy.

Renal Biopsy

It has already been emphasized that the pathology of glomerular disease can often be established only by biopsy. Even though knowledge of the pathology does not always influence treatment it is valuable for assessing prognosis. The enormous enhancement of our understanding of glomerular disease in the last 20 years and the advances that have been made in specific therapy have largely resulted from the widespread use of biopsy. That is not to say that biopsy is necessary in every case; the specific indications vary according to the clinical picture and are given later (see page 59).

Technique

Open biopsy is rarely required as adequate tissue for histological diagnosis can be obtained in most patients by percutaneous needle biopsy. The technique must be learnt from an experienced operator and practised under supervision.

A split needle of the Silverman type with Franklin modification or a disposable 'Tru-Cut' needle (Travenol Laboratories, Inc.) (Figure 10) is usually used. Biopsy is carried out with the patient in the prone position on a firm surface with a small rolled up towel under his abdomen. The preferred site is the centre of the lower pole of the kidney. This is away from major renal blood vessels and the calyces and helps to ensure that the specimen will consist mainly of cortex. The left kidney is usually chosen since biopsy on the right sometimes produces a specimen of liver instead, which is of little value in most renal diseases! The kidney is located by means of an intravenous urogram or by ultrasound. In the former case the site is marked on the skin by reference to bony landmarks—the lower border of the 12th rib and the lumbar spinous processes (Figure 11). With ultrasound the site can be marked directly.

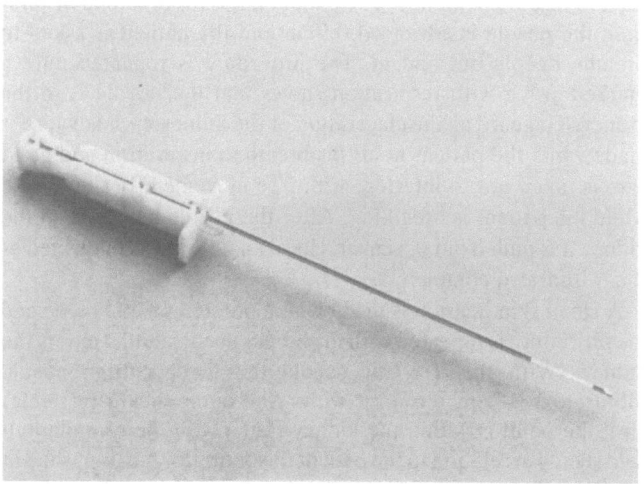

Figure 10. *Disposable 'Tru-Cut' needle, courtesy of Travenol Labs.*

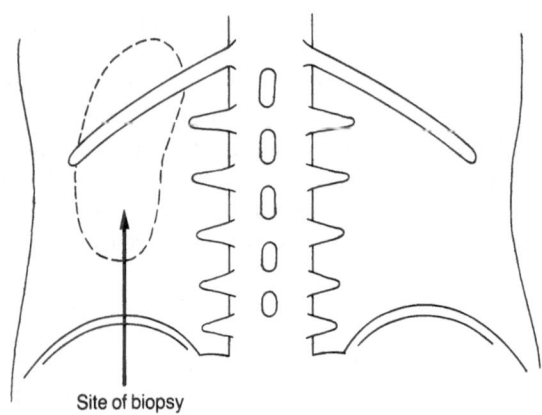

Site of biopsy

Figure 11. *Location of site of kidney biopsy. Patient prone.*

Local anaesthetic is used for most adults, but a general anaesthetic may be required for small children. After infiltration of the skin and subcutaneous tissues, a 10 cm exploring needle is used to locate the kidney. The patient holds his breath in inspiration, the needle is advanced 0.5 cm and the patient is asked to breathe deeply out and in. The procedure is repeated until a marked swing with respiration shows that the needle is in the kidney. To guard against laceration of the kidney each advance is made while the patient holds his breath in inspiration and great care is taken not to interfere with free movement of the needle while the patient is breathing. After the needle has reached the kidney it is pulled out 0.5 cm and local anaesthetic is infiltrated as it is withdrawn completely.

A small skin incision is made with a pointed scalpel blade and the procedure is repeated with the biopsy needle until it enters the kidney. With the Tru-Cut needle the inner cutting needle (obturator) is kept retracted within the outer sheath (cannula) until the point is within the kidney. Then with the cannula hub held steady in relation to the patient the obturator hub is pushed in firmly so that the specimen notch is advanced into the kidney. Next the cannula is pushed sharply down over the obturator to cut off the specimen while the obturator hub is held still. Finally, the needle assembly is withdrawn while the cannula is kept closed over the obturator to retain the specimen within the notch.

Postoperatively the patient is confined to bed for 24 hours, the pulse and blood pressure are recorded at hourly intervals for four hours, then four-hourly for 24 hours, and the urine is closely observed for gross haematuria.

The cylinder of tissue usually contains 10 to 30 glomeruli. The skilled operator has a success rate of well over 90 per cent in properly selected patients.

Complications

Local pain may occur after biopsy and is usually not severe; adequate analgesia should be given and the patient observed carefully. The important complication is bleeding, which may be into the perirenal tissues or into the pelvicalyceal system. In the former case the patient complains of pain and a loin swelling may be found, as well as the circulatory signs of haemorrhage; in the latter case there is heavy haematuria, and clot retention may develop. In either situation, if bleeding continues after blood transfusion and sedation, exploration of the kidney must be carried out. Nephrectomy is very rarely required. A rare but important late complication is the development of an intrarenal traumatic arteriovenous aneurysm (Figure 12), which may cause hypertension. It is suggested by a bruit over the kidney and is confirmed by renal arteriography.

The reported mortality of the procedure is very small. In one review of the literature only 17 deaths were found in more than 10,000 biopsies (White 1963).

Contraindications

The operator must always bear in mind that there is a small but significant possibility of loss of the biopsied kidney so he must be sure of an adequate kidney on the other side. Thus contraindications to percutaneous needle biopsy include a solitary kidney or a major structural abnormality of the opposite kidney. In chronic renal failure of more than moderate severity (creatinine clearance

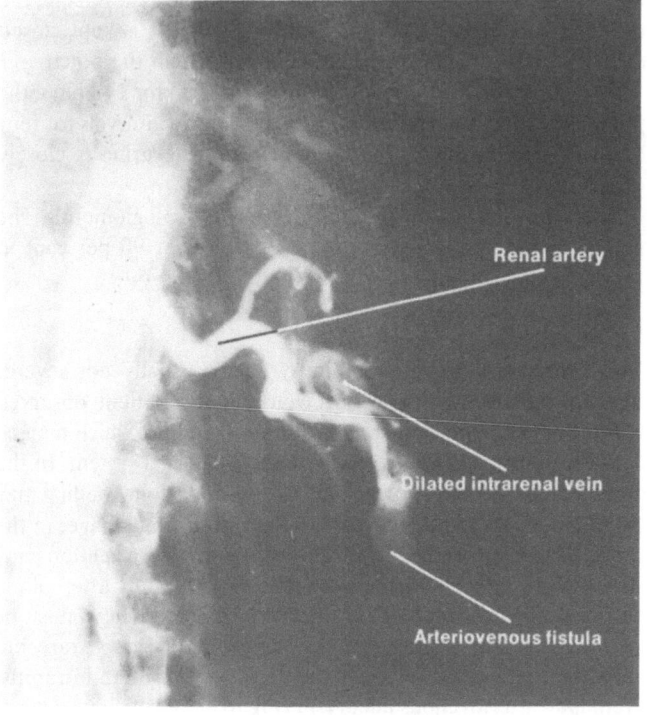

Figure 12. *Intrarenal arteriovenous fistula due to kidney biopsy. Selective left renal arteriogram.*

less than 20 ml/min), biopsy is generally not undertaken since loss of one of the kidneys may reduce the renal function below that necessary to sustain life. An abnormal bleeding tendency is an absolute contraindication. This includes thrombocytopenia, coagulation defects, uncontrolled uraemia or severe hypertension. Small kidneys should not be biopsied as it is difficult to obtain a specimen, the histology is often difficult to interpret, and, in any case, it is unlikely to provide information of therapeutic significance.

Limitations

Considering that the kidneys contain some two million glomeruli and the average renal biopsy contains perhaps 20, it is remarkable that the technique produces such useful information. Nevertheless, the sampling error must always be borne in mind, and biopsy is generally unhelpful in localized lesions of the kidney such as chronic pyelonephritis. Even in the glomerular diseases some glomeruli may be affected and not others, so that the appearance should always be interpreted with caution, especially if the biopsy is a small one.

The other major limitation is the non-specificity in our present state of knowledge of many of the pathological appearances.

7. Pathological Bases of Clinical Syndromes and Indications for Biopsy

Patients present to the doctor with symptoms and signs and not clutching a report on their kidney histology. Therefore it is important to know something about the frequency of the different pathological states underlying the various syndromes. This knowledge will enable renal biopsy to be avoided in many instances.

Even though many large series of renal biopsies have been reported, reliable figures of incidence are not available because of a lack of a uniform nomenclature, both for the syndromes and for the pathology. Also, these series are usually from specialized units, which deal mainly with patients referred from other hospitals, so there is bound to be a bias in selection of cases in favour of those with more severe or difficult disease. Table 4 lists the more common histological changes found in each syndrome in approximate order of their frequency. In most cases meaningful figures of incidence are not available.

Asymptomatic Proteinuria

A small amount of protein in the urine may be a manifestation of any renal glomerular disease or of many other lesions of the kidney and lower urinary tract. If the protein excretion is less than 1 g/24 hr, there are no other abnormal clinical features, no hypertension, no abnormality of the urine deposit, renal function is unimpaired, and the intravenous pyelogram is normal, renal biopsy is often normal or only shows trivial abnormalities. Thus in these circumstances it is not necessary to carry out a biopsy routinely.

Table 4. Pathological basis of the clinical syndromes.

Asymptomatic proteinuria
No or minor non-specific abnormality
Early stage or mild form of any renal disease

Recurrent isolated haematuria (children)
Normal light microscopy or mild mesangial proliferation or sclerosis (mesangial IgA disease)
More serious proliferative glomerulonephritis

Acute nephritic syndrome
Acute diffuse exudative glomerulonephritis (post-streptococcal)
Mesangiocapillary glomerulonephritis
Proliferative with extensive crescents
Systemic lupus erythematosus
Polyarteritis nodosa
Henoch–Schönlein syndrome

Nephrotic syndrome
Primary renal disease
    Proliferative glomerulonephritis—all forms
    Minimal change disease
    Membranous nephropathy
    Focal hyalinosis
Multisystem disease
    Amyloid
    Systemic lupus erythematosus
    Diabetes
    Quartan malaria
    Renal vein thrombosis
    Bee stings
    Mercurials
    Syphilis
    Troxidone
    Constructive pericarditis
    Others

Acute renal failure
Diffuse proliferative exudative glomerulonephritis
Proliferative with extensive crescents
Goodpasture's syndrome
Polyarteritis nodosa
Systemic lupus erythematosus

Chronic renal failure
Mesangiocapillary glomerulonephritis
Proliferative glomerulonephritis with extensive crescents
Membranous nephropathy
Focal hyalinosis
Multisystem diseases

Some patients have an early stage of a more serious glomerular disorder, but here the histology may be difficult to interpret and prognosticate from. Long-term retrospective studies have shown that, in many cases, asymptomatic proteinuria of minor degree is a benign disorder, although the patient should always be followed up. Orthostatic proteinuria is usually benign but it can be a manifestation of organic renal disease.

A problem faced by some of these patients is a socioeconomic rather than a medical difficulty. They may be rejected from certain occupations or have difficulty in obtaining life assurance on account of it. In these circumstances biopsy may be warranted.

In summary, biopsy of a patient with asymptomatic proteinuria is *not* needed unless:

1. Proteinuria is greater than 1 g/24 hr, or

2. Other manifestations of renal disease are present, or

3. There is a non-medical reason for attempting to get a more accurate prognosis.

Recurrent Isolated Haematuria

In the absence of structural abnormality of the urinary tract, of proteinuria, hypertension, or impairment of renal function, recurrent isolated haematuria is also a benign condition in most cases. Particularly if the haematuria is intermittent and in children, biopsy is not required, except sometimes to reassure anxious parents. It is naturally important to be certain that the blood is not coming from a renal tumour or from a lesion of the lower urinary tract. In children an IVU often suffices but adults will need cystoscopy as well. The presence of bloody or granular casts in the urine is a useful indication that the bleeding is from the renal parenchyma. If doubt remains, a biopsy should be performed since, even though no definite glomerular abnormality may be found, red blood cells may be seen in Bowman's space or the tubules, confirming the renal origin of the blood.

It will be seen in Table 4 that focal glomerulonephritis is not listed among the histological causes in children. In the past the term has been used almost synonymously with recurrent haematuria, but, in fact, it is found much more frequently in other clinical settings.

In some cases a history of haematuria is obtained in other members of the family. This form of familial renal disease should not be confused with the syndrome of hereditary nephritis and deafness (Alport's syndrome), which has a much more sinister prognosis.

Thus, in general, biopsy in recurrent isolated haematuria is *not* needed unless:

1. Other manifestations of renal disease are present, or

2. It is necessary to confirm that blood is coming from the kidney, or

3. To reassure parents.

Acute Nephritic Syndrome

A patient presenting with the classical features of acute post-streptococcal nephritis nearly always has the diffuse exudative lesion, and biopsy is not required as a rule. More sinister conditions, however, occasionally present with the sudden onset of haematuria and proteinuria, and may be difficult to differentiate. The combination of the nephrotic syndrome with haematuria nearly always indicates a more serious underlying cause. The persistence of proteinuria or abnormality of the urinary sediment even for several months are not in themselves indications for biopsy.

In general biopsy in the acute nephritic syndrome should *not* be carried out unless:

1. Oliguria persists for more than a few days, or

2. Renal function remains significantly impaired or deteriorates, or

3. Serum C3 concentration remains subnormal after six weeks, or

4. Nephrotic syndrome exists in combination with haematuria.

The Nephrotic Syndrome

The nephrotic syndrome has many causes and biopsy is often needed. However, it is often possible to distinguish the minimal change lesion without the aid of a biopsy, and it is particularly desirable to avoid this since most of the sufferers are children. If the typical features of minimal change are present, a trial of steroid therapy can be given and biopsy carried out only if there is no response.

In the multisystem disorders the diagnosis is often made from the extrarenal manifestations of the disease, but biopsy may still be valuable for prognosis.

Biopsy in the nephrotic syndrome *should* be carried out unless the following conditions apply:

1. Age two to ten years.
2. No hypertension.
3. No haematuria.
4. No significant impairment of renal function.
5. Highly selective proteinuria.

Acute Renal Failure

Most patients with acute renal failure have acute tubular necrosis, and the only common glomerular cause is acute post-streptococcal glomerulonephritis, which is usually transient. There are, however, more sinister causes, so biopsy is sometimes needed.

Biopsy in acute renal failure should *not* be carried out unless:

1. No precipitating factor of acute tubular necrosis is apparent.
2. Renal tract obstruction has been excluded.
3. Oliguria persists for more than a few days.

Chronic Renal Failure

Glomerular disease is the most important cause of chronic renal failure, but when renal function is severely impaired it is of little more than academic interest to ascertain the cause since treatment for the renal lesion is not available. Furthermore, the kidneys are often shrunken so that biopsy is technically difficult, and the histology of the kidney is difficult to interpret.

Biopsy in chronic renal failure *should* be carried out unless:

1. A structural abnormality of the kidney or renal tract is demonstrated by radiology or urological examination.

2. The kidneys are reduced in size, or

3. Creatinine clearance is less than 20 ml/min.

8. Treatment

There are two main lines of treatment of renal glomerular disease:

1. Symptomatic.
2. Treatment of the renal lesion.

Symptomatic treatment is designed to correct the disturbance of function brought about by the kidney disease. The nature of the treatment depends on the clinical disturbance irrespective of the underlying pathology, and in general it has no influence on the course of the pathological process. On the other hand the choice of treatment aimed at the renal lesion depends entirely on the nature of the lesion and not on the clinical features.

It follows that different criteria are used to measure the efficacy of each line of treatment. Symptomatic treatment is assessed by its effect on such factors as the patient's symptoms, the degree of oedema and the blood urea, in so far as it is altered by non-renal mechanisms. However, criteria of response to treatment of the renal lesion are objective measurements of renal function such as 24-hour urine protein excretion, creatinine clearance, and occasionally follow-up renal biopsy.

Symptomatic Treatment

Asymptomatic Proteinuria

No treatment is available or necessary for asymptomatic proteinuria but when (as in most cases) the underlying lesion is considered to be a benign one, the patient should be reassured accordingly. He should be assisted in any difficulty regarding employment or life assurance, but since it is not possible to be entirely certain of the prognosis in any individual case he may still be unacceptable in certain jobs, for example, as a commercial airline pilot.

Long-term follow-up is necessary, both in the patient's interests in case the lesion turns out to be the earliest stage of a progressive disease, and in order to further our knowledge of the natural history. However, once the condition is seen to be stable, follow-up should be at long intervals, that is, six months or one year, to prevent the patient becoming too preoccupied with his kidneys.

Isolated Haematuria

Here again reassurance of the patient or his parents is of prime concern. Exacerbations are often provoked by minor upper respiratory tract infections, and long-term antibiotic prophylaxis is sometimes prescribed. But the infections are usually viral and the value of antibiotics in most cases is dubious.

Acute Nephritic Syndrome

During the oliguric phase management is the same as for other varieties of acute renal failure, with restriction of fluid, protein and salt intake. The volume of fluid given each 24 hours is based upon the previous day's urine output with an additional allowance of 400 ml (in adults) for insensible losses. Calories are given in the form of pure carbohydrate, such as glucose drinks, Hycal and sweets. Since the duration of oliguria is usually brief there is no need for a very high calorie intake, or for an allowance of protein. The rare patient with oliguria of more than a few days duration will need dialysis, at which time the diet can be liberalized. As the urine output increases the fluid intake is correspondingly increased and the diet derestricted. Penicillin is given for 10 days to eliminate any remaining streptococci. The patient is kept in bed until diuresis is established and the signs of circulatory overload have disappeared. There is no evidence that there is any value in more prolonged bed rest.

The above measures suffice for most patients, but when complications occur they must be treated energetically. Pulmonary congestion with symptoms or acute pulmonary oedema should be treated with intravenous frusemide. Large doses may be needed and if an initial dose of 20 mg is ineffective, repeated injections should be given, doubling the dose each time until diuresis ensues. Venesection is effective, but rarely necessary with the use of frusemide. Digitalis is of little value unless there is some unrelated cardiac disorder.

Uncomplicated hypertension does not require treatment until the diastolic blood pressure is above 110 mm Hg. Any oral antihypertensive agent may be used, but for a hypertensive crisis a parenteral preparation is needed, such as hydrallazine 20 mg i.v. or diazoxide 300 mg i.v. Encephalopathy must be controlled quickly by lowering the blood pressure and by using diazepam for fits. If pulmonary oedema or hypertensive encephalopathy does not respond promptly to the above measures there should be no hesitation in using peritoneal dialysis, which is effective treatment for both complications.

Patients with persisting oliguria should be treated by dialysis when the blood urea reaches 40 mmol/l (plasma creatinine 900 μmol/l) or sooner if there is serious hyperkalaemia or any other indication. Though most of these patients fail to recover renal function, one or two do, so dialysis should be continued for several weeks even if there is no possibility of transfer to a maintenance dialysis or transplantation programme.

Nephrotic Syndrome

The object of treatment in the nephrotic syndrome (Table 5) is to relieve the oedema. A very low salt diet is useful but unpalatable and with modern diuretics it is not usually necessary. Moderate restriction of sodium intake to 40 mEq/day is all that is required in most cases. A high protein intake is of some help in maintaining the serum albumin concentration, but since it is difficult to give much protein without salt there is little to be gained by an intake of more than 80 g/day.

Diuretics are the mainstay of treatment. Thiazides, such as bendrofluazide 5 to 20 mg daily, suffice for milder cases, but more

Table 5. Management of the nephrotic syndrome.

Dietary sodium restriction—40 mEq/24 hr
High protein intake—80 g/24 hr
Thiazide diuretics—bendrofluazide 5 to 20 mg daily
Potassium supplement—Slow-K 6 tablets daily
Aldosterone-antagonist diuretics—spironolactone
100 mg b.d.
Frusemide—40 to 2,000 mg daily
Human plasma protein fraction i.v.

resistant ones will need frusemide or ethacrynic acid. If there is poor renal function as well as the nephrotic syndrome, very large doses may be required. However, it is very important to avoid too precipitate a diuresis because this can cause severe hypovolaemia in nephrotic patients, who often have a reduced circulatory volume even before treatment. Frusemide 40 mg should be given on the first day and the dose doubled each day until diuresis occurs. The effect is assessed more reliably by weighing the patient daily than by measuring the urine output. A weight reduction of 1 kg/day (less in children) is the most that should be allowed. A daily dose of frusemide of 1 g or more is sometimes needed, and may be given safely by this means. Frusemide is available in 500 mg tablets.

The intravenous infusion of protein only has a transient effect on the serum albumin concentration as it is rapidly excreted. Nevertheless, it is of value in initiating the diuresis and in protecting the patient against hypovolaemia when diuretic treatment is instituted. Human plasma protein fraction may be used instead of the very expensive salt-poor human albumin, because concurrent diuretic therapy will eliminate the sodium given in the plasma. Plasma protein infusions should be used in severely oedematous small children and in adults with resistant oedema or with signs of pre-existing hypovolaemia, such as postural hypotension. It is important to avoid dehydration, especially in patients with impaired renal function, since this may be further compromised. It is often safer to leave these patients with a little ankle oedema than to attempt to rid them of all excess fluid.

Supplementary potassium is needed, often in large amounts. The quantity contained in the combination diuretic–potassium tablets is usually insufficient and the supplement should be given separately as Slow-K or Kloref, six or more tablets daily. The addition of spironolactone (200 mg daily) potentiates the action of other diuretics, and aids in conserving potassium. Invasive methods of removing fluid such as acupuncture and paracentesis are virtually never required today.

Nephrotic patients are prone to infection, which must be treated early, vigorously and with specific agents.

In addition, patients may be unduly susceptible to ischaemic heart disease as a result of their hyperlipidaemia. Treatment has been advocated with a low cholesterol and saturated fat diet, high intake of polyunsaturated fat and agents such as clofibrate. The value of such treatment has not yet been established .

Acute and Chronic Renal Failure

Management of acute and chronic renal failure is beyond the scope of this book (see *Acute and Chronic Renal Failure*, Boulton-Jones 1980). However, one point deserves mention, and that is the treatment of hypertension complicating chronic renal failure. Hypertension occurs in many patients with chronic glomerular disease, and hypertensive vascular damage is often a very important factor contributing to further deterioration in renal function. In the past it has been taught that lowering the blood pressure would aggravate uraemia, but it has now been demonstrated convincingly that control of hypertension slows down decline of renal function, unless renal failure is far advanced. A precipitous drop in blood pressure may temporarily raise the blood urea and must be avoided, but long-term smooth control of hypertension is essential.

Treatment of Renal Lesion

The only drugs of proven value in the specific treatment of glomerular disease are corticosteroids and cytotoxics, but even these are useful only in very limited circumstances. Many other drugs are under investigation, but none is as yet established as beneficial.

Cytotoxic Drugs and Corticosteroids

Cytotoxic drugs and corticosteroids suppress antibody formation and interfere with immunological reactions at other stages as well. Both also inhibit the inflammatory reaction and platelet aggregation. Bearing in mind the pathogenetic mechanisms of glomerular disease, all these actions gave grounds for hope that the drugs would be of value in therapy. Earlier uncontrolled observations supported this optimism, but controlled trials since have given equivocal results. The solitary condition in which treatment produces undisputed and consistent benefit is the minimal change lesion. Paradoxically, here there is little evidence of an immunological pathogenesis and none at all of inflammation or cell proliferation.

The drugs are also of value in many cases of lupus nephritis, but in all other varieties of progressive glomerular disease there is no consistent benefit.

Anticoagulants

Deposits of fibrin probably play an important part in glomerular damage in some forms of rapidly progressive glomerulonephritis. Animals can be protected from experimental nephritis by depleting them of fibrin or by pretreatment with anticoagulants. Good results have been claimed for the use of anticoagulants in human disease, but patients with very severe lesions and oliguria rarely respond. Heparin is probably more effective than warfarin and is usually used in conjunction with steroids, cyclophosphamide, and the platelet stabilizer dipyridamole. More experience is needed before the value of this treatment is established.

Toxic Effect of Drugs

The toxic effects of steroids, cytotoxic drugs and anticoagulants are numerous, serious and potentially lethal. They are sufficiently well known not to need reiterating here. However, one danger of cyclophosphamide that has only recently been emphasized is the possibility of permanent sterility.

The use of these drugs should therefore be considered with great care when their value is dubious, as in most cases of renal glomerular disease. One controlled trial of prednisone in the nephrotic syndrome has actually shown a higher mortality in the treated group than in the controls (Black et al. 1970). There is a considerable temptation to use them in the more serious progressive varieties of disease in an attempt to forestall the otherwise inevitable development of end stage renal failure. But it must be remembered that, now that dialysis and transplantation can be offered to many patients, end stage renal failure does not necessarily mean death. Patients may be denied the potential benefits of these forms of treatment as a result of death from drug toxicity.

The practical aspects of treatment are considered separately for each group of conditions.

Plasma Exchange

A novel approach to the treatment of glomerular disease caused by immune complexes or by autoantibodies is to remove the offending agent from the circulation by means of plasma exchange. This technique also depletes humoral mediators of injury, such as complement and fibrinogen. Immunosuppressive drugs are given at the same time. A 'cell separator' machine is used to exchange several litres of plasma for plasma protein fraction. Access to the circulation by means of an arteriovenous shunt enables the procedure to be repeated at frequent intervals.

Most of the patients treated so far have had either Goodpasture's syndrome or another variety of rapidly progressive (crescentic) nephritis. Improvement occurred in most of those who had some residual renal function when treatment was started.

Minimal Change Lesion

Virtually all patients with minimal change disease respond to steroids, which should be given to all those who are symptomatic. Proteinuria disappears and all manifestations of the disease remit. If there is no response within four weeks, the diagnosis is likely to be wrong and renal biopsy should be carried out. An initial dose of 60 mg daily of prednisone is used and the dose is gradually reduced over eight weeks. About 50 per cent of patients remain in permanent remission, but the remainder relapse after stopping treatment. It is these patients who present difficulty in management. A second course of prednisone may be followed by a sustained remission, but most of these patients continue to relapse whenever the drug is withdrawn. After the second relapse an attempt is made to find the smallest maintenance dose of prednisone which will keep the urine free from protein. If this is low, long-term maintenance treatment is given. If the dose is high, the patient runs a serious risk of steroid toxicity, which in children includes permanent stunting of growth. It is in this group of 'persistent relapsers' that cyclophosphamide treatment is considered.

Cyclophosphamide produces remissions as regularly as steroids and it has the advantage that the remissions are more often permanent or long-lasting after cessation of therapy, even in those who relapsed persistently after steroids. About half the patients remain free from proteinuria at two years. Because of the possibility of permanent sterility, careful consideration should be given before cyclophosphamide is used in children or adults of reproductive age. Nevertheless, when prolonged high dose steroid therapy is the only alternative and steroid side effects are manifest, its benefits outweigh the dangers and it should be given. The optimum course of treatment is probably 3 mg/kg body weight for eight weeks.

Systemic Lupus Erythematosus

Immunosuppressive drugs have a favourable effect on the renal manifestations of many patients with systemic lupus erythematosus and they improve the long-term prognosis of those with diffuse proliferative disease. The current evidence supports the use of a combination of prednisone with cyclophosphamide, or azathioprine rather than steroids alone.

Other Multisystem Diseases

The value of immunosuppressive drugs in polyarteritis, Goodpasture's syndrome and Henoch–Schönlein disease has not been defined by controlled trials. However, spectacular successes are obtained in some patients, particularly if renal failure is not too advanced, and a trial of prednisone and cyclophosphamide should be given in progressive cases.

Severe Proliferative Glomerulonephritis with Extensive Crescents

Several systematic though uncontrolled trials have shown impressive results from the use of an anticoagulant/immunosuppressive 'cocktail' comprising prednisone, azathioprine, dipyridamole, and heparin or warfarin (Kincaid-Smith et al. 1968; Cameron et al. 1975). Again, improvement is rare in patients already anuric or severely oliguric when treatment is begun. This potentially lethal combination of drugs needs very careful supervision and the patients often require a period of dialysis, so that treatment is best given at a specialized renal unit.

Membranous Nephropathy

The value of treatment is very difficult to assess in this very chronic disease with its substantial spontaneous remission rate. Most trials have shown no definite benefit but one controlled study of alternate day high dosage prednisone has demonstrated a significant difference between treated and untreated patients with respect to reduction in proteinuria and preservation of renal function (Glassock 1978).

Mesangiocapillary Glomerulonephritis

Treatment with an anticoagulant–immunosuppressant cocktail appears to have benefited some patients, but no controlled trials have yet been completed.

Focal Glomerulosclerosis

Although a small proportion of steroid-responsive patients have been reported in some trials, this lesion, in general, is not helped by immunosuppressive treatment.

Acknowledgements

I am very grateful to Dr David Turner for the electron photomicrographs, and to Mr Rodney Machling for many of the histological preparations.

References

General

Boulton-Jones, A., *Acute and Chronic Renal Failure*, 1980, Update Books, London, Topic Pack Series.

Chapter 1

Ellis, A., *Lancet*, 1942, **i**, 1.

Chapter 4

Sharpstone, P., Ogg, C. S. and Cameron, J. S., *Br. Med. J.*, 1969, **2**, 533.

Chapter 6

White, R. H. R., *Arch. Dis. Child.*, 1963, **38**, 260.

Chapter 8

Black, D. A. K., Rose, G. and Brewer, D. B., *Br. Med. J.*, 1970, **3**, 421.
Cameron, J. S., Gill, D., Turner, D. R., Chantler, C., Ogg, C. S., Vosnides, G. and Williams, O. G., *Lancet*, 1975, **ii**, 923.
Glassock, R. J., *Proc. VIIth Int. Cong. Nephrol.*, Karger, Basel, p. 425.
Kincaid-Smith, P., Saker, B. M. and Fairley, K., *Lancet*, 1968, **ii**, 1360.

Further Reading

Historical

Bright, R., *Reports of Medical Cases*, Longman, Rees, Orme, Brown and Green, London, 1827.

Volhardt, F. and Fahr, I., *Die Brightsche Nierenkrankheit*, Springer, Berlin, 1914.

Longcope, W. T., *J. Clin. Invest.*, 1936, **15**, 277.

Ellis, A., *Lancet*, 1942, **i**, 1.

Addis, T., *Glomerular Nephritis: Diagnosis and Treatment,* MacMillan, New York, 1949.

General

Kincaid-Smith, P., Mathew, T. H. and Baker, E. L., *Glomerulonephritis, Morphology, Natural History and Treatment*, Wiley, New York, 1973.

Pathology

Heptinstall, R. H., *Pathology of the Kidney,* Little, Brown and Co., Boston, 1974.

Pathogenesis

Peters, D. K. and Williams, D. G., in *Recent Advances in Renal Disease,* N. F. Jones (Ed.) Churchill Livingstone, Edinburgh, 1975, p. 90.

Treatment

Cameron, J. S., *Br. Med. J.,* 1977, **1**, 1457.

Membranous Nephropathy

Pierides, A. M., Malasit, P., Morley, A. R. *et al.,* Quart. J. Med., 1977, **46**, 163.

Focal Glomerulosclerosis

Habib, R., *Kidney Int.,* 1973, **4**, 355.

Systemic Lupus Erythematosus

Baldwin, D. S., Gluck, M. C., Lowenstein, J. *et al., Am. J. Med.,* 1977, **62**, 12.

Henoch-Schönlein Syndrome

Meadow, S. R., Glasgow, E. F. White, R. H. R. *et al., Quart. J. Med.,* 1972, **41**, 241.

Amyloidosis

Triger, D. R. and Joekes, A. M., *Quart. J. Med.,* 1973, **42**, 15.

Diabetic Nephropathy

Watkins, P. J., Blainey, J. D., Brewer, D. B. *et al., Quart. J. Med.,* 1972, **41**, 437.

Asymptomatic Proteinuria

Levitt, J. I., *Ann. Int. Med.,* 1967, **66**, 685.

Recurrent Haematuria

Roy, L. P., Fish, A. J., Vernier, R. L. *et al. J. Pediat.,* 1973, **82**, 767.

Nephrotic Syndrome

Black, D. A. K., Rose, G. and Brewer, D. B., *Br. Med. J.,* 1970, **3**, 421.
White, R. H. R., Glasgow, E. F. and Mills, R. J., *Lancet,* 1970, **i**, 1353.
Cameron, J. S., Chantler, C., Ogg, C. S. *et al., Br. Med. J.,* 1974, **4**, 7.

Post-streptococcal Glomerulonephritis

Baldwin, D. S., *Am. J. Med.,* 1977, **62**, 1.

Mesangiocapillary Glomerulonephritis

Habib, R., Kleinknecht, C., Gubler, M. C. *et al., Clin. Nephrol.,* 1973, **1**, 194.

Rapidly Progressive Glomerulonephritis

Beirne, G. J., Wagnild, J. P., Zimmerman, S. W. *et al., Medicine (Baltimore)*, 1977, **56**, 349.

Index